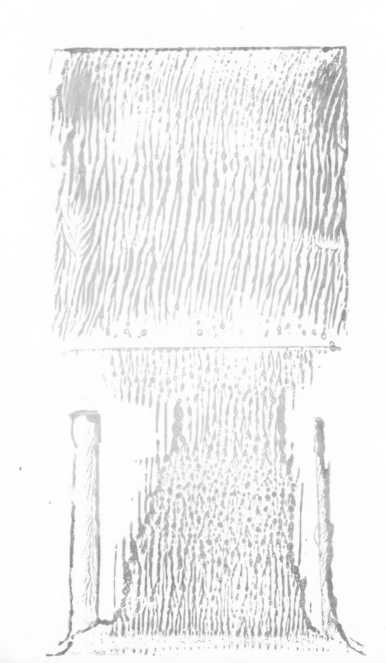

Living With Diabetes

Living With Diabetes

THE REVOLUTIONARY SELF-CARE DIABETES PROGRAM
DEVELOPED BY
ROCKEFELLER AND CORNELL UNIVERSITY
RESEARCHERS

Genell J. Subak-Sharpe

WITH INTRODUCTION AND AFTERWORD BY
DRS. CHARLES M. PETERSON AND LOIS JOVANOVIC,
CO-MEDICAL DIRECTORS,
DIABETES SELF-CARE PROGRAM

JAMES V. WARREN, M.D.
FRONTIERS IN MEDICINE
CONSULTING EDITOR

DOUBLEDAY & COMPANY, INC.
GARDEN CITY, NEW YORK
1985

Library of Congress Cataloging in Publication Data
Subak-Sharpe, Genell J.
Living with diabetes.

Bibliography: p. 269
Includes index.
1. Diabetes. 2. Self-care, Health. I. Title.
RC660.S83 1985   616.4'62   84–13622
ISBN: 0-385-18769-6

To Angela, Bob, Jim, Rayna, and Wendy

Acknowledgments

Many people are involved in the writing of a book and this one is no exception. Simply listing all the people who have provided invaluable information and insight into what is involved in diabetes self-care would take up several pages. While it is not possible to recognize all of them, there are those who contributed so much it would be derelict not to at least mention their names. They include Barbara Turro, R.D., the Diabetes Self-Care Program dietition who has been extraordinarily helpful in preparing the dietary sections of this book. Other program staff members who worked with me include Karen Wauchop, Lorraine Lerner, Anne Grant, Andy Boston, Faye Ettinger, and Ann Duckles.

This book would not have been possible without the diligence and help of Drs. Charles Peterson and Lois Jovanovic, Co-Medical Directors of the Diabetes Self-Care Program. Not only did they make available important information about diabetes self-care, they also shared their special insight about what is involved in coping with the disease. Katharine Alling, director of the Diabetes Education Foundation in Rochester, N.Y., also has been particularly helpful.

Perhaps the greatest contribution, however, came from the Diabetes Self-Care Program patients who openly discussed the many problems of living with diabetes and also shared their triumphs. Many of these accomplishments—having a healthy baby, pursing a chosen career, traveling abroad, going to school—are things many of us take for granted, but for a person with diabetes, they are proof of extraordinary effort and constant attention to controlling vital body processes.

Dr. James V. Warren, the Consulting Editor for the Frontiers in Medicine series, has been an invaluable partner in the writing and editing of this manuscript. My Doubleday editors, Loretta Barrett, Felecia Abbadessa, and Susan Sandler, deserve particular credit for their patience and sensitive, meticulous editing. I also want to thank

Andrea Rainer, the medical illustrator who prepared the drawings for the book, and Emily Paulsen, who helped with research, typing, and myriad other tasks.

Finally, special thanks to my husband, Gerald, and children David, Sarah, and Hope Subak-Sharpe for their understanding and patience.

Foreword

The past decade has provided tremendous hope to people with diabetes mellitus. It has become clear that elevated blood sugar levels are toxic to the body. However, it has also become possible to maintain blood sugar levels in the normal range. A number of techniques and tools are now available to help patients with diabetes take charge of their own blood sugar and fix it.

The process is not an easy one. We have found that both patients and professionals require about forty hours of training to learn the principles and skills of controlling blood glucose levels. The author has invested more than eighty hours learning about diabetes, first in a diabetes self-care program for patients and then in a Cornell course for health professionals. These two programs have formed the basis for this book.

The proof of the book's value will be the lowered blood sugar levels of the people with diabetes who follow its advice and the improved understanding of their family and friends. So get to work and good reading!

Lois Jovanovic, M.D.
Charles M. Peterson, M.D.
Co-Medical Directors,
Diabetes Self-Care Program

Contents

PART III: PROBLEM SOLVING

PART IV: TYPE 2 DIABETES

Introduction

When people talk about major diseases, heart attacks and cancer usually head the list, followed by some of the relatively rare disorders like muscular dystrophy that capture public attention with telethons and other fund-raising drives that bring in millions of dollars and an outpouring of sympathy for their victims. Compared to these headline diseases, diabetes is relatively neglected, even though it is one of the most serious health problems in this country. At least ten million Americans have diabetes, and it is estimated that another ten million people have the disease without knowing it. For reasons that are not completely clear, the incidence is increasing by about 6 percent a year, meaning that the number of people with the disease will double in about fifteen years.

The economic and medical effects of diabetes are profound. The disease is directly responsible for about 40,000 deaths a year, but when deaths from diabetic complications such as vascular disorders and kidney failure are added, the figure soars to 300,000. This makes diabetes the third leading cause of death in the United States, exceeded only by heart disease and cancer. Diabetes is also the major cause of new cases of blindness. More than 80 percent of all amputations in this country are performed because of diabetes. It is a leading cause of kidney disease and also increases the risk of both heart attacks and strokes. People with diabetes spend more time in the hospital, require more drugs, and see their doctors more often than the general population. Their total medical bill is estimated at more than $10 billion a year.

Many popular misconceptions about diabetes persist, both in the general public and among many physicians and other health professionals. There is a popular belief, for example, that diabetes can be easily controlled: all the person with the disease needs to do is take a shot of insulin every day and not eat sweets and he or she can lead a normal life. At the other extreme, many people still believe that diabetes is hopeless no matter what is or is not done. The fact is, diabetes is a disease about which there are still many unanswered questions, but tremendous advances of the last few decades are making it possible for an ever-increasing number of people with the disease to lead normal, productive lives and to achieve common objectives that were unthinkable only a few years ago. For example, a growing number of young women with diabetes are becoming mothers. Until recently, it was highly unusual for a diabetic woman to achieve pregnancy, and very few of those who did get pregnant were able to deliver normal, healthy babies.

With proper management, there are few things that the person with diabetes cannot do. But no one should be lulled into thinking that living with diabetes is simple. Effective control requires understanding the disease and knowing how to anticipate and solve problems, preferably before they occur. Contrary to popular belief, a person with diabetes can eat an occasional ice cream cone or piece of pie, but doing so without problems requires knowing how to match insulin and food. You don't have to be a dietitian to master the technique, but you should understand the metabolic differences between carbohydrates and protein and know how to calculate grams of each when they appear on your plate.

In researching this book, dozens of people with diabetes were interviewed. Repeatedly, they described feelings of being controlled by the disease and its treatment, and often without the desired results. One person recalled:

When I first got diabetes, I went to a famous diabetes clinic. I was put on a strict schedule and diet. I was told exactly how much insulin I needed to take each day and at what time I had to take it. I had to eat six meals a day, whether I was hungry or not, and I was told exactly how much and at what time I could exercise. And I was told that if I didn't follow the instructions to the letter, terrible things would happen to me. I tried as hard as I could to live by the rules, and terrible things happened anyway. After a while, I sort of devised my own devices to keep from having an insulin reaction or having my blood sugar go out of sight. But I never felt that I was in control. Life was a constant mood swing and I usually felt lousy. After a few years, I accepted that this was what it meant to have diabetes. But then I began to have eye and kidney problems, and I knew that if I didn't try something else, I would end up blind and dead before I was thirty-five. I was living by the rules, but they weren't helping.

Time and again, I listened as patients described their frustration and confusion, their feelings of rejection and inability to cope. One young man, who is now a third-year medical student, recounted his recurring torture of going to summer camp:

My parents were determined that I live a normal life, so they sent me to camp with my friends. The camp director and medical people knew that I had diabetes, so taking my insulin was not a problem. But our daily schedule called for an hour's swim before lunch. After a few minutes, I could feel myself getting weaker and weaker. Each time, I would feel sure I wouldn't make it. I tried stuffing myself with crackers before swimming, but this wasn't enough. Now I realize that the exercise was poorly timed, and that it should have come after lunch or at a time when my blood sugar was high enough to carry me through.

This is but one of hundreds of examples of the kinds of problems a diabetic patient encounters in living with the disease. Fortunately, modern diabetes therapy has developed systems to achieve the kind of control and flexibility that would allow this young man to swim with his fellow campers and not experience the dangerously low blood sugar he remembers only too well.

This book is intended to give people with diabetes the understanding and guidance they need to control their diabetes, not vice versa. It is based on a pioneering program in diabetes self-care that was developed by physicians and researchers at Rockefeller University and the Cornell University Medical College. The Diabetes Self-Care Program, widely recognized as the most comprehensive and innovative treatment regimen of its kind, is designed not only to teach you all you need to know about the disease but also how to evaluate your lifestyle and mold your treatment to accommodate it. "All too often, patients are told they must live their lives according to their disease and treatment program," says Dr. Lois Jovanovic, one of the Diabetes Self-Care Program's medical directors, who herself has diabetes. "Our goal is to teach you how to adapt your treatment to your life, yet at the same time achieve a better degree of diabetes control."

The Rockefeller-Cornell Diabetes Self-Care Program embraces several basic principles of managing the disease. Patients are expected to learn and practice home blood glucose monitoring—a relatively simple, two-minute self-test to measure the amount of sugar in a drop of blood. Multiple injections of insulin are favored for most patients instead of a single daily shot. Specific insulin doses are determined by a number of factors, including blood sugar levels, the amount of food that is to be consumed, and the level of physical activity. Patients are also taught how to adjust insulin dosage for special circumstances, such as infection or illness or, for women, the premenstrual phase of the monthly cycle. There is also a special program for the diabetic woman who is or is planning to become pregnant.

This book is not intended to replace or alter the advice of your personal physician. But it will give you the background information needed to follow your doctor's instructions and to achieve better control of your diabetes. If you do not now monitor your own blood glucose or are not on a regimen that employs the principles described in the following chapters, you might want to ask your doctor if the concepts embodied in the Diabetes Self-Care Program might be appropriate for you. If your doctor is not familiar with the program, show him or her this book, or you can seek additional information by contacting the program directors at 344 East 63rd Street, New York, N.Y. 10021. While the information in this book was gathered with the permission of the Diabetes Self-Care Program and the author has attended classes sponsored by the program for both patients and health professionals, the writing and presentation of material are solely the work of the author, who is not in any way affiliated with the program, Rockefeller or Cornell Universities, or National Medical Care, Inc., program managers.

Living With Diabetes

I

Type 1 Diabetes and Its Control

The Basics of Diabetes

Diabetes is a chronic disease affecting many body systems and functions, particularly those concerned with metabolism, the processes by which the body converts food into forms that can be used for energy, growth, or to meet other body needs. A person with diabetes, for example, is unable to use, or burn, blood sugar (glucose), the body's fuel for the brain, muscles (including the heart), red blood cells, and other body tissues. Glucose is also needed to utilize other foods. As a result, as diabetes advances, the patient enters a state of starvation, no matter how much he or she eats. To better understand what happens in diabetes, let us take a brief look at the processes and organs involved.

Diabetes is the most common of the endocrine disorders, a family of diseases caused by a malfunction of one or more endocrine glands. A gland is defined as any part of the body that produces a secretion. There are two broad categories of glands: the exocrine, which send their secretions through a duct (or ducts) for external use, and the endocrine, whose secretions go directly into the bloodstream for internal use. The exocrine system includes the glands that produce saliva, milk, and sweat; the endocrine glands produce the various sex hormones, adrenaline, cortisone, the thyroid hormones, and insulin, among others. In diabetes, the problem lies in the pancreas, the gland in which insulin, as well as a number of digestive juices, is manufactured. Diabetes can result either from insufficient insulin or an inability of the body to use it. Insulin is produced by specialized cells called the islets of Langerhans, named for the scientist who discovered them.

Although these clusters of cells, which are scattered throughout the pancreas, were discovered many years ago, insulin was not discovered until 1921, when two Canadian scientists, Drs. Frederick G. Banting and Charles H. Best, isolated it from animal pancreas glands.

The major function of insulin is to regulate the amount of glucose that circulates in the blood. Almost all carbohydrates and about 50 to 60 percent of all protein is converted into glucose by the digestive process. Glucose that the body does not immediately need is stored, mostly in the liver, as glycogen, which is released and converted back to glucose as the body needs it. After a meal, about 90 percent of the carbohydrates passes through the liver, where 55 to 60 percent is stored as glycogen and the rest is released into the blood as glucose. Most of this glucose is used by the brain and red blood cells; the remainder is metabolized by the muscle and fat tissue. Any rise in blood glucose is sensed by the pancreas, which responds by secreting extra insulin. This insulin aids in glucose metabolism by the muscle and fat tissue. It also enhances the liver's storage of excess glucose as glycogen and inhibits the liver from releasing glucose until the amount already circulating in the blood is used. In this way, insulin helps control the level of blood glucose. When there is not enough insulin or when the body is unable to use its insulin effectively, there is a buildup of glucose in the blood, a condition called hyperglycemia. As the body becomes overloaded with glucose, some of the excess will be secreted by the kidneys into the urine.

Insulin also has an important effect on fat metabolism. The fat consumed in a meal is stored in triglycerides in the adipose, or fat, tissue. Some of the excess carbohydrate calories are also used to form the triglyceride molecule, a process that requires insulin. Insulin helps prevent the breakdown of triglycerides from the adipose tissue; when these adipose triglycerides are metabolized in the liver, ketones, which are highly acidic substances, are formed. Some of these ketones can be used by the muscles and other peripheral tissues, but when the body is overloaded with ketones, the excess will accumulate in the blood and spill over into the urine. In the absence of insulin, excessive fatty tissue is broken down by the liver, with a resulting buildup of ketones. (Complications of this situation will be discussed in later sections.)

experience of the program developers. They stress, however, that each patient requires individualized supervision by a physician, preferably one experienced in treating diabetes. The principles and examples cited in this book work for most patients, but each patient has individual differences that require a physician's expertise and medical judgment. Thus, the information in this book should not be used to change your treatment regimen without first discussing it with your doctor.

DIFFERENCES BETWEEN
TYPE 1 AND TYPE 2 DIABETES

Characteristic	Type 1	Type 2
Age of onset	Usually during first three decades of life, especially during periods of rapid growth	Usually after forty, increasing with age
Precipitating factors	Altered immune response to certain viruses (?)	Obesity, pregnancy, infection, and other stresses
Endogenous insulin	Little or none	May be normal, high, or low
Fasting blood glucose	High	May be near normal
Carbohydrate intolerance	Severe	Moderate to severe
Response to fasting	High blood glucose	Blood glucose becomes normal
Response to insulin	Normal	May be resistant
Response to diet alone	Negligible	Usually marked
Response to oral hypoglycemic drugs	None	Usually good

Adapted from C. J. Goodner, "Newer Concepts in Diabetes Mellitus, Including Management." *DM*, September 1965, p. 19. Copyright © 1965, Year Book Medical Publishers, Inc., Chicago.

How Diabetes Is Diagnosed

Diabetes, like most diseases, has certain symptoms that point to its diagnosis. In fact, the major symptoms of diabetes have been well known by doctors for hundreds of years. As early as 1500 B.C., ancient doctors described the classic symptoms of diabetes. These early physicians named the disease diabetes mellitus because of its major early symptoms: "diabetes" is from the Greek word for fountain or syphon, referring to the copious urination that is a common sign, and "mellitus" is from the Latin word for honey, since the urine has a sickly sweet smell and taste. In fact, the earliest diagnostic test for diabetes involved smelling and tasting the urine for the telltale sweetness caused by an overflowing of blood sugar or glucose into the urine.

Diabetes should be suspected in anyone who suddenly begins experiencing excessive, almost insatiable thirst, copious urination, hunger, and loss of weight. Other symptoms include weakness, fatigue, mood swings, and increased vulnerability to infection, particularly vaginal infections in women. Leg cramps or pins-and-needles sensations in the legs also may occur in diabetes. Diabetes may cause male impotence. Eye problems, such as blurred vision and hemorrhages of the tiny blood vessels of the retina, are still other signs of diabetes, although these usually do not occur until a more advanced stage of the disease.

Sometimes these symptoms may be ignored until the approach of diabetic acidosis, a result of buildup of too much blood sugar that the body cannot metabolize and a breakdown of body fat and other tissue, leading to an accumulation of ketones, acidic substances. Dentists

sometimes alert a patient to the early stages of ketoacidosis, as the
condition is known, because it causes a fruity, sweetish breath odor.
Diabetic acidosis is a potentially life-threatening situation characterized by tremendous thirst, weakness, dryness of the skin and tongue,
and nausea and vomiting. If untreated, this can progress to diabetic
coma and death.

Not everyone with diabetes experiences noticeable symptoms; it
is estimated that perhaps as many as half of all people with diabetes,
or nearly ten million Americans, may have some form of diabetes and
not know it. Most of these undiagnosed patients fall into the type 2
category, in which the pancreas continues to produce insulin. This
insulin production may be insufficient to meet the body's needs or
there may be adequate insulin but the body is failing to fully use it.

In people without symptoms, a doctor may be alerted to the
possibility of diabetes by a urine test that shows the presence of sugar,
or glycosuria. But sugar in the urine is not always a sign of diabetes; in
some people, glycosuria may simply mean the kidneys are unable to
handle large amounts of blood sugar and are excreting some into the
urine. Also, many people with mild diabetes do not "spill" sugar, or do
so erratically. Thus, the definitive diagnosis must be based on the
presence of excessive sugar in the blood.

Several measurements of blood sugar may be required before a
diagnosis of diabetes can be made. In people with type 1 diabetes, in
which the pancreas is producing little or no insulin, the diagnosis is
usually straightforward. A blood sample is taken early in the morning,
before any food has been consumed, a test called a fasting blood
glucose. If two separate fasting blood glucose tests are positive, meaning that there is more than 140 milligrams of glucose per deciliter of
blood (mg/dl), or 7.8 millimoles in the new terminology, the diagnosis
of diabetes is established. In borderline cases, in which the fasting
blood glucose is 105 to 140 mg/dl, additional testing may be necessary
if there are symptoms that suggest diabetes. (If there are no symptoms, such as thirst, increased urination, or weight loss, and no family
history of the disease, further testing probably is not necessary.) People who fall into this borderline group may be asked to undergo periodic blood sugar measurements, and if they are overweight, to go on a

weight-reduction diet. If they are sedentary, they also may be advised to increase their exercise because physical activity helps the body burn excess blood glucose.

If further diagnostic workups are required, they probably will include a glucose tolerance test as well as a complete physical examination and medical history (see Patient Medical History Form at end of chapter). As the name implies, a glucose tolerance test is designed specifically to measure the body's response to a sugar or glucose challenge. To make sure that the test results are not skewed by abnormal conditions, a person undergoing a glucose tolerance test must follow specific instructions for several days before the test. For example, some people may think they will "do better" on the test if they cut back on food, especially sweets, or lose weight before taking it. This can produce a false positive result. If you do not have diabetes, the more carbohydrates, especially sugar, you eat, the harder the pancreas works to produce insulin. If you suddenly stop eating or cut back on carbohydrates, the pancreas does not have to function at its full capacity. Then when challenged with a large amount of sugar, as during the glucose tolerance test, it will be unable to meet the demand and blood sugar will be abnormally high, leading to a diagnosis of diabetes. However, if you had eaten normally in the few days before the test, the pancreas would have been able to meet the glucose challenge. This is why doctors should instruct people undergoing a glucose tolerance test to consume at least 100 to 150 grams of carbohydrates a day for the three preceding days.

Lack of exercise also can influence the outcome of a glucose tolerance test. People who are hospitalized or confined to bed before taking it will have higher blood glucose levels than normally active individuals. This explains why older people or those suffering from other illnesses sometimes have abnormal glucose tolerance tests even though they do not have diabetes. Certain illnesses, especially liver disease, also may produce abnormal test results.

Several medications can alter glucose tolerance; your doctor or the laboratory administering the test should be aware of any drugs you may be taking. Drugs that are known to alter test results include diuretics (water pills), which may be prescribed for high blood pressure or edema (the accumulation of body fluid); synthetic estrogens, such as those found in birth control pills; glucocorticoids, or steroid drugs, which are prescribed for a number of inflammatory and other conditions; and Dilantin, an anticonvulsive drug often prescribed for people with seizure disorders.

These drugs work in different ways to alter glucose tolerance; therefore, various measures may be taken to counter their effects. For example, diuretics, especially those in the thiazide class, tend to lower the body's level of potassium. In turn, potassium depletion hinders the release of insulin in response to glucose. This can be overcome by administering a potassium supplement before performing a glucose tolerance test. Steroid drugs are strong insulin antagonists, and when they are given the pancreas responds by increasing its output of insulin. This effect may persist for months after stopping the drug; therefore, an abnormal glucose tolerance test in someone who has been on steroids is not necessarily an indication of diabetes. The same effect is encountered with synthetic estrogens. Dilantin has a direct effect on the insulin-producing beta cells and thereby inhibits insulin production. This effect usually ceases when the drug is stopped.

Another drug that may produce abnormal glucose tolerance test results is large amounts of nicotinic acid, which may be taken to lower high cholesterol. Excessive use of alcohol may impair glucose metabolism and alter test results. Finally, some drugs, such as large amounts of salicylates (aspirin) or monoamine oxidase (MAO) inhibitors, which are sometimes prescribed to counter depression, may produce false negative results because they may lower blood glucose. Doctors advise that people on MAO inhibitors stop taking them at least a month before undergoing a glucose tolerance test.

Pregnancy is still another factor that alters glucose tolerance. Since the fetus requires some of the maternal blood sugar, the mother's fasting glucose levels tend to be somewhat lower than usual. In addition, a woman's use of glucose is slowed during pregnancy, meaning that the blood sugar levels may be somewhat high in the later stages of a glucose tolerance test. To compensate for these natural changes, different criteria are used for evaluating a glucose tolerance test during pregnancy.

Patients who have undergone ulcer or other gastric surgery also have altered carbohydrate metabolism. To avoid false results, the glucose challenge should be administered intravenously rather than orally.

THE TEST ITSELF

The test itself is rather simple. It is usually done on an outpatient basis, often in a clinic or doctor's office. A blood sample is taken to measure your blood glucose, which should be in the high or borderline range of 105 to 140 mg/dl. You then swallow a drink containing 75 mg of glucose, and your blood glucose is measured hourly over the next three hours. There is considerable disagreement over the interpretation of results and the exact criteria for a diagnosis of diabetes. The Cornell-Rockefeller doctors use the following criteria, which are based on standards provided by the National Diabetes Data Group. If blood glucose is 200 mg/dl or higher an hour after the sugar drink is swallowed and remains at that level for the next two hours, the test is considered positive for diabetes. Measurements of less than 200 but more than 165 mg/dl at one hour, 145 mg/dl at two hours, and 125 mg/dl at three hours are considered borderline, or indicative of impaired glucose tolerance. Blood glucose measurements below these levels are in the normal range. The urine also may be tested for sugar at the same time the blood samples are taken; however, as noted earlier, the presence or absence of sugar in the urine is not an accurate diagnostic tool in diabetes.

Even so, these results are not always definitive. As stressed by Dr. Mayer Davidson of UCLA and author of the textbook *Diabetes Mellitus: Diagnosis and Treatment,* "Although abnormal glucose tolerance clearly delineates a group of subjects who may eventually manifest overt diabetes mellitus, only a minority of these individuals will do so. An approximately equal number of this group will have a normal result in subsequent tests." In studies involving several hundred patients, 5.3 percent of 588 who had normal test results eventually developed diabetes, most of them ten to twenty years later. Only 22.9 percent of the 401 who had positive tests went on to develop overt symptoms of diabetes, usually within five years. Overt diabetes is most likely to develop in people whose blood glucose is in the 200 mg/dl range after two and three hours and those who have other risk factors, such as a strong family history of diabetes, are over the age of fifty, and are overweight.

SUMMING UP

A number of symptoms arouse the suspicion of diabetes, but diagnosis entails having an abnormally high blood glucose level. Diagnosis is easiest in type 1 diabetes, in which the pancreas is secreting little or no insulin. Two or more fasting blood glucose measurements, taken in the morning before any food has been consumed, of 140 mg/dl or higher indicate diabetes. In borderline cases or type 2 diabetes, in which there is still suspicion of possible diabetes even though the fasting blood sugar level is normal or high but not in the diabetic range, further testing may be in order. This usually involves one or more glucose tolerance tests in which the pancreas is challenged by having the patient consume a large amount of sugar and then monitoring its effect on blood glucose.

A number of factors, including diet, level of physical activity, general health, pregnancy, and the use of certain drugs, can alter test results. Even a positive glucose tolerance test does not necessarily mean that the person has diabetes or is likely to develop it in the near future. In addition, taking positive preventive steps at this stage, such as losing excess weight and increasing physical activity, may prevent the development of overt diabetes. In any event, a strong suspicion of diabetes is a warning to watch for further symptoms and to see a doctor promptly if the condition appears to be progressing.

PATIENT MEDICAL HISTORY FORM

Please complete this form as accurately as possible
(use other side if additional space is needed)

Date:
Name:_____
Address:_____
_____

Home phone #_____
Occupation:_____
Business address:_____
_____

Business phone #_____
Medical insurance (type):_____

Other
Sex (check one): M___ F___   Race: Black___ White___ (specify)_____
Date of birth:_____   Place of birth:_____

Marital status:_____   Name of spouse:_____
Business address:_____
Business phone #_____

Referring private physician:_____
Address:_____
Phone #_____

Please state briefly why you wish to be seen at the Diabetes Self-Care Program (include any signs or symptoms you may have at this time): _____
_____
_____
_____

Have you ever experienced these symptoms of high blood sugar?

	Yes	*No*	*When did these symptoms appear?*
1) frequent urination	___	___	
2) drinking large amounts of water	___	___	
3) severe hunger	___	___	
4) blurred vision	___	___	
5) frequent urinary and/or vaginal tract infections	___	___	
6) uncontrolled rapid weight loss	___	___	

Have you ever experienced these symptoms of low blood sugar?

	Yes	*No*	*When did these symptoms appear?*
1) profuse sweating	___	___	
2) rapid heart rate (at rest)	___	___	
3) pallor (loss of facial color)	___	___	
4) light-headedness	___	___	
5) fainting	___	___	

Have you ever been hospitalized for ketoacidosis/high blood sugar?
Place_____ Date(s)_____ _____
Have you ever been hospitalized for hypoglycemic shock?
Place_____ Date(s)_____ _____

Date onset of diabetes:_____
Do you or have you ever used pills to control your diabetes?   Yes___   No___
Name of medication_____
Date when started_____   Dose___   How often_____

If you are using insulin, list:

Type	Amount	Time of day taken

Are you currently taking any other medications? Please list:

Medication	Dose	How often taken

List any sleeping pills or tranquilizers that you are currently taking, and how often.

_____

_____

What is your favorite alcoholic beverage? _____
How much do you drink: per day___   per week___   per month_____

Immunizations: Please check the following if known:

Tetanus, last booster—at age	Not known	(Other)
DPT completed—at age	Not known	(Other)
Polio completed—at age	Not known	(Other)
Smallpox—at age	Not known	(Other)
Measles—at age	Not known	(Other)
Rubella—at age	Not known	(Other)
Mumps—at age	Not known	(Other)

(Past history continued)
Allergies, please list the ones known:_____
Type of reaction:_____

Food:
Drug:
Penicillin given, reaction:
Other:

Infections

	Yes	No	Date (if known)
Measles	___	___	_____
Mumps	___	___	_____
Chicken pox	___	___	_____
Scarlet fever	___	___	_____
Hepatitis	___	___	_____

Ophthalmologic

Do you wear glasses?   Yes___   No___   Since_____

Do you wear contacts?   Yes___   No___   Since_____

When were your eyes last checked?_____

Were you informed of any eye problems?_____

    Retinal artery occlusion?   Yes___   No___

    Hemorrhaging?   Yes___   No___

    Double vision?   Yes___   No___

    Blurred vision?   Yes___   No___

Have you ever received laser treatment?   Yes___   No___   Date_____

Have you ever had eye surgery?   Yes___   No___   Date_____

Auditory

Have you ever experienced hearing
difficulties?   Yes___   No___   Date_____

Do you wear a hearing aid?   Yes___   No___   Date_____

When was the last time your hearing was checked?_____

Nasal

Do you have frequent nosebleeds?   Yes___   No___

Dental

When was your last dental exam?_____

Do you frequently get cavities?   Yes___   No___

Are you prone to infections in the
mouth?   Yes___   No___

Cardiovascular   *Yes   No   Date(s)*
Have you ever had:
  Chest discomfort   ___ ___ _____
  Heart attack   ___ ___ _____
  Rapid heart rate   ___ ___ _____
  Irregular rhythm   ___ ___ _____
  Rheumatic fever   ___ ___ _____
  Swelling of the ankles   ___ ___ _____
  Cramping/pain in the legs   ___ ___ _____
Do you have high blood pressure?   ___ ___ _____

Respiratory
Do you smoke?   ___ ___
If yes, how much?   _____
Do you have a chronic cough?   ___ ___ Since____
Have you ever had:
  Tuberculosis   ___ ___ _____
  Pneumonia   ___ ___ _____
  Blood in your sputum   ___ ___ _____
  Asthma   ___ ___ _____
  Bronchitis   ___ ___ _____
Most recent chest X ray or tine test   _____

Gastrointestinal
Have you ever had an ulcer?   ___ ___ _____
Do you frequently experience nausea
or vomiting?   ___ ___ _____
Have you ever vomited blood?   ___ ___ _____
How many bowel movements do you have a day? _____
Has blood ever been present in stool?   ___ ___ _____
Have you experienced:
  Frequent diarrhea   ___ ___ _____
  Frequent constipation   ___ ___ _____
Do you have difficulty digesting fatty foods?   ___ ___

Genitourinary   Yes   No   Date(s)

Have you ever experienced:

   Blood in your urine   ___ ___ _____

   Painful urination   ___ ___ _____

   Frequent urination at night   ___ ___ _____

   Spilling protein in your urine   ___ ___ _____

Reproductive

Have you ever contracted:

   Syphilis   ___ ___ _____

   Gonorrhea   ___ ___ _____

   Other venereal diseases   ___ ___ _____

Have you experienced:

   Impotence   ___ ___ _____

   Infertility   ___ ___ _____

Complete if female:

Menses—onset age:

   Flow: Minimal___ Moderate___ Heavy_____ Pads/day___

   Discomfort: Minimal___ Moderate___ Severe_____ None____

   Frequency: Every___days Regular____ Irregular____

   Duration: Days_____ Last menstrual period_____ Other____

Pregnancies: Total_____ Full-term___ Premature___

   Multiple births_____ Abortions___ Now alive___

Contraception used_____ Last Pap test_____

Neurologic   Yes   No   Date(s)

Have you had:

   A stroke   _____ _____ _____

   Balance problems   _____ _____ _____

   Numbness and tingling in your

   extremities   _____ _____ _____

   Seizures   _____ _____ _____

Do you have frequent headaches?   _____ _____ _____

Do you have frequent dizzy spells?   _____ _____ _____

Do you have frequent tremors?   _____ _____ _____

Neurologic (continued)   *Yes*   *No*   *Date(s)*

Have you ever sought psychological
consultation?   _____   _____   _____

If so, for what reasons?_____

_____

_____

Family History

   Mother: Alive_____ Deceased_____ Age/age at death_____
   General health: _____

_____

   Father: Alive_____ Deceased_____ Age/age at death_____
   General health: _____

_____

Do (did) either of your parents
have heart disease?   Mother_____ Father_____ Neither_____

Do (did) either of your parents
have diabetes?   Mother_____ Father_____ Neither_____

Siblings:

   Name   *Sex*   *Age*   *General health*
1. _____   _____   _____   _____
2. _____   _____   _____   _____
3. _____   _____   _____   _____
4. _____   _____   _____   _____

Do (did) any of your siblings have heart disease? How many?_____

Do (did) any of your siblings have diabetes? How many?_____

Are there any other members of your family with diabetes?

If so, please list: _____

_____

_____

The Diabetes Self-Care Program

People with diabetes require considerably more medical care than the average person. Not only do they have to keep the diabetes itself under control, but they also are more vulnerable to an assortment of other health problems, such as infections, circulatory disorders, kidney trouble, heart disease, eye problems, and nerve disorders. Not all diabetic patients develop these complications, but they should have frequent medical checkups and pay attention to warning signs. Obviously, finding a physician with whom the patient and his or her family have good rapport is important. Fortunately, most people with diabetes have access to a center or physician well versed in its treatment. In this era of ever-increasing medical specialization, it is not surprising that there are so many clinics, internists, endocrinologists, or other physicians specializing in diabetes. Most large teaching hospitals or medical centers also have special clinics for diabetes. Many diabetic patients go to several doctors or clinics before settling on a regimen that seems to work well for them. Those who do quickly learn that not all these centers or specialists agree on the precise details of diabetes management, which may be confusing for the patient but is understandable in a disease in which there are so many variables and unknowns.

While having good, reliable medical care is vital for the person with diabetes, in the final analysis it is the patient who must manage the disease. A doctor or other health professional can instruct and prescribe, but it is up to the individual patient to do what needs to be done to keep blood glucose under control and thereby lead a better life. With experience, many people with diabetes learn to do this very well. But large numbers either find that their therapeutic regimens are impossibly difficult to reconcile with their lives or simply do not work for them. This is why the self-care program developed by Cornell-Rockefeller researchers was selected from among the many other clinics or centers as the focus of this book. Giving the individual diabetic the knowledge and skills he or she needs to control the disease is the primary objective of the Self-Care Program. Patients who have been through the intensive one-week course or women who have "graduated" from the pregnancy program with healthy, long-desired babies attest to its success. Many patients who enroll in the program are surprised to learn that they can adjust their own insulin dosage to allow more flexibility in their lives. They learn how to use food and exercise to help control blood sugar and how to handle potentially dangerous situations.

Patients are not the only ones who can benefit from the program. Doctors, nurses, and other medical personnel who have taken the course for health professionals agree that they have acquired new knowledge about diabetes management and, just as importantly, have gained new insight into what life with the disease is like from a patient's perspective.

In this book, you will meet some of the physicians who have been instrumental in developing the program, as well as many of the other health professionals who are experts in such areas as nutrition, exercise, and specialties related to complications of diabetes. You will also meet patients who are representative of the broad spectrum of people with the disease, ranging from rebellious adolescents to extraordinarily diligent and motivated expectant mothers.

The Diabetes Self-Care Program evolved from the work of a group of diabetes researchers at two sister institutions in New York City: Rockefeller University and The New York Hospital-Cornell Medical Center. The researchers, principally Drs. Charles M. Peterson, Lois Jovanovic, and Robert Jones, have collaborated on a number of studies on various aspects of diabetes for nearly a decade. But in addition to studying the scientific aspects of the disease, all have been devoted to helping patients live better lives by showing them how to achieve control of diabetes. As co-medical directors of the Diabetes Self-Care Program, Drs. Peterson and Jovanovic demonstrate a special kind of caring that patients respond to almost instantly. One, a thirty-five-year-old college professor, describes it this way: "Dr. Jovanovic came to see me when I was a patient at New York Hospital. I was having kidney problems and I had developed high blood pressure. Instead of trying to tell me not to worry, that everything was going to be okay—a line I had heard from doctors ever since I was seven years old—she said: 'This disease is a real bummer that sometimes scares me half to death.' That was what I had been feeling for years, but no doctor had ever come right out and said it to me. I later learned that she had diabetes herself and knew what she was talking about; she also knew exactly how I felt at that moment."

While Dr. Jovanovic may know from her personal experience that diabetes is no joke and thereby impart a special understanding, little time is wasted on self-pity. "Diabetic patients can be very manipulative," she says. "We learn early on that the disease is an acceptable excuse for everything from temper tantrums to failing a test. But our mission here is to turn our lives around and to gain control over the disease. This takes concentration and a lot of work and there are still going to be times when things go wrong. But if we can figure out why certain things are happening, then we have a better chance of preventing them in the future."

The Diabetes Self-Care Program draws heavily on the resources of the nearby Rockefeller University and Hospital and The New York Hospital-Cornell University Medical Center and is often referred to as the Rockefeller-Cornell Diabetes Program. Patients come from all over the country, sometimes referred by their own doctors, sometimes at the suggestion of friends, former patients, or others who have heard of the innovative program. Most can achieve their objective in an intensive week, during which they are at the center from 8:30 A.M. through the dinner hour. The time is spent learning by doing: mastering measuring their own blood glucose levels; measuring the effects of certain foods and exercise on those levels; learning how to match food and insulin with a kind of precision that most doctors don't know; sharing their experiences and emotional responses with their fellow patients. A good deal of the time is spent in a classroomlike setting, listening to lectures from noted authorities in various fields of medicine related to diabetes. And, as would be expected, enrollment in the program also entails a complete physical examination, including an exercise stress test.

In preparing this book, the author went through a typical course with a group of five patients. Names have been changed to protect their privacy, but all agreed to share their experiences.

The five range in age from twenty-seven to forty and all have type 1 diabetes. Two had known each other briefly when they were in high school; the others were meeting for the first time. At first glance, the group's initial gathering could be mistaken for any adult education seminar or class. All five look healthy; you'd never pick one of them out of a crowd and say, "This person has a potentially life-threatening disease." On this first day of the program, all have arrived early and are seated around a table in the center's lecture room. There's a slide projector, chalkboard, and other familiar classroom objects; on the table is an assortment of supplies used in testing blood glucose. The five, although attentive, also seem a bit apprehensive while waiting for Dr. Jovanovic, who is to give the opening lecture at 9 A.M. As one of the nurses draws small amounts of blood from each patient, the five chat quietly among themselves, each telling what has brought him or her here.

Bob, a thirty-five-year-old professor from an upstate New York university, has had diabetes since he was seven years old. His sister also has the disease, and he fears he will develop the complications that have left her nearly blind and with neuropathy, a disease affecting the nerves, in her feet and legs. His doctor has assured him that his diabetes is in "good control" and that he is doing all the right things: measuring his own blood sugar, adhering to a diet, exercising regularly. Still, he has developed high blood pressure and early signs of kidney disease. He has suffered several hemorrhages of the tiny blood vessels in his eyes and has undergone laser treatments to try to minimize the damage; even so, he has diminished peripheral vision and is terrified by the prospect of losing his eyesight. Bob also worries about being able to continue supporting his wife and two children. "I guess I've come here out of a sense of desperation," he confesses. "My doctor keeps telling me not to worry, that I'm doing fine. But I know this isn't true."

Jim, a twenty-seven-year-old stage manager, shares Bob's concerns. He too developed diabetes when he was seven and has also had eye hemorrhages and kidney problems. Recently married, he wants to spare his wife worry over his health. Unlike Bob, whose job gives his life a regular schedule and security, Jim's profession is full of uncertainties. Jobs tend to be short-lived, highly demanding for a few days, weeks, or months, and then he is back looking for another show or film. He cannot keep the regular hours advocated by most diabetes specialists: meals may be skipped or eaten on the run; one job may involve working at night, the next may have day hours or a split shift of morning rehearsals and an evening performance. "I've never been able to make my life fit my treatment," he says. "When I heard that this program can fit my treatment to my life, I decided to give it a try." He hopes to go on an insulin pump—a small, computerized device that delivers small amounts of insulin throughout the day and can also be used to administer larger doses as needed to handle food intake. He is somewhat apprehensive about trying something new, but he knows that Dr. Jovanovic uses an insulin pump herself and he is eager to at least give it a try.

Connie also wants to go on an insulin pump. She has been through the Self-Care clinic's intensive pregnancy program and is one of Dr. Jovanovic's real success stories. "I never thought I would be able to have a baby," Connie relates. "I had never had regular periods and even though my doctor said my diabetes was in good control, I never felt healthy." Connie was diagnosed as having diabetes when she was fourteen. She married shortly after graduating from high school. "All my life I wanted to be a mother, but I had thought my diabetes had ruled that out. Then I began hearing about this program and a study being done by Dr. Jovanovic on pregnancy and diabetes." With the support of her husband, Connie decided to volunteer as a patient in Dr. Jovanovic's pregnancy research project. This involved spending some time in the hospital in an intensive effort to bring her diabetes under very tight control and to learn what would be involved in maintaining that kind of control through pregnancy. Women participating in this study were required to keep their blood glucose in the normal range for three months before attempting pregnancy. "At first, it was like having another full-time job," she recalls, "but I never felt better in my life. I started having regular periods and I looked and felt healthy." After meeting the necessary criteria, she soon found she was pregnant.

Connie's pregnancy was a lot of work. She had to monitor her blood glucose seven or eight or more times a day and meticulously adhere to her treatment program. But she was rewarded with an absolutely perfect six-and-a-half-pound full-term baby girl, Amy. "I could never have done it without the support and help of my husband," Connie tells the others. Obviously, both feel that the effort was worthwhile; Connie is now back in the program to learn how to use an insulin pump in hopes of another pregnancy. "Amy is now almost two years old, and both my husband and I want another baby. But Amy takes so much of my time, I don't think I can manage her and at the same time pay as much attention to my diabetes as I did during my first pregnancy." She hopes that mastering an insulin pump will remove some of the time and effort required in controlling her diabetes. Like Jim, she is a bit frightened at the prospect: "I know I can keep my diabetes under control with injections, but what if something goes wrong with the pump?" Still, as Dr. Jovanovic likes to point out, "It's hard to find a more motivated patient than a diabetic woman who wants to have a baby. They'll do almost anything to protect that baby. . . ." Connie is eager to do whatever is necessary to repeat her feat with Amy.

Alice, a twenty-seven-year-old secretary, has had diabetes since she was eight. She admits she has been a bit casual about the disease. At present, she takes one injection of insulin a day—a mixture of Regular and a slow-acting one. "I'm hungry all the time," she confesses, and she often yields to the temptation of rich foods. "When I want to lose weight, my doctor has told me I can just cut back on my insulin a bit and spill a little sugar," a piece of advice that makes Dr. Jovanovic shudder because it runs contrary to the current philosophy of the tighter the blood glucose control, the better for the patient.

Spilling sugar would mean that Alice's glucose level is so high the body is trying to get rid of the excess by excreting it in the urine. In effect, when this happens Alice is in a state of starvation, even though she may be eating all sorts of rich foods, because her body is unable to properly metabolize the food.

Alice has been married for two years, and she and her husband are eager to have a family. So far, her attempts to become pregnant have been unsuccessful; she has come to the Diabetes Self-Care Program not only to learn a better method of controlling her disease, but also in hopes of entering the center's pregnancy program.

Rita is an executive with a car-leasing firm. Although she has type 1 diabetes, she did not develop the disease until she was in her thirties. She sums up her reason for enrolling in the program by saying, "I'm totally out of control and I don't know what to do about it." Her blood glucose fluctuates widely, a fact she confirms with self-testing. "I've gained fifteen pounds in the last six months. I follow my doctor's instructions to the letter and still, I seem to be going from bad to worse."

Promptly at eight forty-five, Dr. Jovanovic arrives, looking more like a pert schoolgirl than a doctor, with her long dark hair worn in a single braid and a brightly colored scarf tied around her waist. She has met many of the patients at earlier interviews and, of course, Connie is an old friend. "Why didn't you bring our baby?" she asks. Dr. Jovanovic takes a very maternal interest in her patients' offspring: dozens of baby pictures decorate her office walls at Cornell, and when asked how many children she has, she replies, "Two of my own and about two hundred of my patients'."

Connie, tall, slim, and attractive, has been concerned that an insulin pump will be conspicuous: "I don't want friends coming up to me in the supermarket asking 'What's that?'," she explains. Dr. Jovanovic, dressed in a fashionable sweater, trim skirt, and boots, has no telltale bulges or tubing to indicate she is wearing an insulin pump. Finally, Connie asks, "Where is it?" Dr. Jovanovic pats the scarf tied around her waist; the pump, about the size of a pack of cards, is tucked in the folds, and the tubing that leads to the syringe implanted in her abdomen also is hidden by the scarf.

Dr. Jovanovic goes around the table, asking each patient to recite his or her morning blood sugar and to review his or her insulin regimens. The group visibly becomes more relaxed as she makes brief comments to each. Then, speaking to all five, she promises a week that is going to be both rewarding and frustrating: rewarding because by its end each one should have blood sugar levels that are in the normal range (something that only Connie can now claim), and frustrating because initially some may actually feel worse. "Most of you have blood glucose levels that are too high," she explains. "Your bodies have become accustomed to the high levels and as these come down, you may feel tired or out-of-sorts. But as your body readjusts to normal blood sugar, you'll begin to feel better physically." She also speaks of the emotional uplift of gaining a sense of control. "Many of you now feel that you are being controlled by your diabetes; by the end of the week, our goal is to have *you*, not your disease, in control."

And so begins what all five later describe as one of the most important and enlightening weeks of their lives. No time is wasted: on that first day, they learn the basic skills of effective self-care. These include such things as how to calculate insulin doses on the basis of body weight and how to match insulin and food. Instead of planning meals around food exchanges, they learn to build their meals around grams of carbohydrates. They also learn to use blood glucose meters, portable machines about the size of a small tape recorder that are used in glucose self-testing.

Over the next five days, these patients will spend ten or more hours a day at the center. They will get to know each other very well and will share both problems and solutions. Since doctors, nurses, or other health professionals are always nearby, they soon begin to lose their fear of experimenting with food, exercise, and other factors that affect blood glucose. By week's end, all will have different insulin regimens and all will have blood sugar levels that are in the normal range. Both Connie and Jim get their insulin pumps and both weather their first experiences of something going amiss. They all learn a new way of matching food and insulin by counting grams of carbohydrates; a system they find easier and more accurate than the food exchanges many had used before. Their problems do not disappear in a single week—far from it. Bob suffers a series of eye hemorrhages that again stir his fear of blindness; Jim has several insulin reactions; Rita and Alice both go through a few days of feeling unwell as their blood sugar levels move down into a more normal range. For Connie, this is something of a refresher course, but she is still a bit apprehensive about managing her diabetes through a much-wanted second pregnancy.

On Friday, as the time for departure nears, several become fearful of again striking out on their own; of putting what they have learned to use without the backup of Drs. Jovanovic or Peterson. Most of the last morning is devoted to an intense group therapy session during which each one describes the anger, frustration, and fear that are always just below the surface. From the session emerge even closer bonds with each other and an enhanced determination to keep fighting. Also, each has Dr. Jovanovic's home telephone number and instructions to call her at appointed times, something they all do over the following weeks.

"Many people come to us with very little understanding of the disease or how to manage it," Dr. Jovanovic explains. "Others are very knowledgeable but are frustrated by a regimen that is not suitable for their lifestyles. Still others are trying very hard to follow their doctors' instructions, but simply are not able to control their blood sugar levels. Our task is to evaluate each situation and then help the individual understand what he or she must do to remedy the situation. It's a big assignment for one week; this is why we want to keep in touch with the patients even after they return home. And some come back for a second session or refresher course. In the end, most people find they can master self-care, often to a degree that both they and their doctors had thought impossible in the beginning."

4

Self-Monitoring,
the Key to Diabetes Self-Care

A typical session at the Diabetes Self-Care clinic begins with the patients gathering around the table in the classroom and quietly assembling the items needed to measure their own blood glucose. Each calmly pricks his or her finger, squeezes out a drop of blood onto a chemically treated strip, and within a couple of minutes each knows his or her level of blood glucose. Although measuring blood sugar has become routine for them and thousands of other people with diabetes, there are still many who do not know how to use this simple technique to control their disease.

For decades, diabetic patients have been taught to monitor their disease, but until recently they lacked the tools to really determine the degree of blood sugar control. Traditionally, home monitoring has involved testing the urine for the presence of sugar and/or ketones, the acidic by-product of fat metabolism. Although urine sugar tests are a useful tool in diabetes management, they are not as accurate or as meaningful as blood glucose measurements because by the time sugar appears in the urine, it usually means that blood glucose has been too high for some time. Also, some people with diabetes do not spill sugar, and others, whose kidneys cannot handle even moderate amounts of glucose, may excrete some sugar even when there is no hyperglycemia. In the words of Dr. Peterson, "At best, urine glucose measurements are a warning signal, but it tends to come too late." Still, for many years this was the only home test available to the diabetic patient; a blood sugar measurement was done only by a doctor or other health professional, and even in a hospital setting, it often took hours to get the results back from a laboratory. And when they had the results, the doctors still did not know whether or not the long-term control of blood sugar was good or poor. The test told them only the level of blood sugar at the time the blood was drawn.

All this has changed dramatically with new tests that measure long-term blood glucose levels and also with the development of easy-to-use kits that enable patients to measure their own blood glucose in just two or three minutes. The test that reveals the state of average blood glucose levels over the previous month or so is based on the principle that high levels of blood glucose affect the red blood cells, particularly the hemoglobin, the component that carries oxygen. Glucose molecules become permanently attached to hemoglobin, altering its structure (a process called glycosylation). Normally, only a small percentage of hemoglobin is glycosylated, which is referred to as the percentage of hemoglobin A_{1C}, or HbA_{1C}. In poorly controlled diabetes, however, the level of glycosylated hemoglobin will be much higher than normal. For example, a hemoglobin A_{1C} of 3 to 6 or 7 percent is considered normal; a hemoglobin A_{1C} of 9 to 12 percent is not unusual in patients with consistently high blood glucose levels. A reading in this range tells the doctor that blood glucose has been higher than normal over the previous month or six weeks. This test has become invaluable in helping physicians gauge the effectiveness of diabetic patients' efforts to normalize blood sugar.

To help patients achieve normal blood sugar, Self-Care Program physicians and other experts increasingly advocate home glucose testing. There are now a number of reasonably priced self-monitoring kits on the market, all operating on the same general principle. The procedure itself is fairly easy, and most people can master it in a day or two.

Supplies needed to measure your own blood sugar include sterile needles or lancets, alcohol swabs, gauze pads or tissues, reagent strips, and a glucose meter. Initially, a doctor, diabetes educator, or other trained health professional should show you how to do the test. You start by assembling all the items in the kit and then washing your hands thoroughly with soap and warm water. Alcohol wipes should not be used before the tests since the substance can interfere with results. Blood is usually taken from a fingertip. Many people feel nervous about sticking their finger with a needle or lancet; there are a number of devices that hold a sterile lancet and can be triggered easily to produce a fast, painless prick. A large puncture is not needed since the test requires only a couple of drops of blood. The sides of the fingers should be used because they are less sensitive than the tips and inner pads, where the nerves are concentrated. To make it easier to get enough blood from a tiny prick, make sure your hands are warm. Squeezing or "milking" the finger for a few seconds before pricking it also stimulates blood flow and makes it easier to squeeze out the needed drops. The first drop should be wiped away with a clean tissue or gauze pad. Many people become nervous and their hands perspire when they do the test, and perspiration may mix with the blood and alter test results.

A small amount of blood is placed on a chemically treated reagent strip. These strips contain an enzyme and a color-generating compound that interact with the blood glucose, causing the treated portion of the strip to change color. The strip can be interpreted visually, matching the color change with the chart that accompanies each bottle. But since the color changes are sometimes difficult to gauge, especially by patients whose eyesight might be affected by diabetes, Self-Care Program physicians urge patients to use a small, portable machine, or glucose meter. Make sure that the reagent strips are compatible with a particular glucose meter and that the machine has been correctly calibrated for the strips. Manufacturers of the various glucose meters provide detailed instructions on how to calibrate them; the sales representatives or diabetes educators also are available to teach the steps involved.

Although the procedures vary somewhat among the different machines, all operate on the principle of bouncing light off the color of the strip and then indicating the level of blood glucose on a digital printer. Some machines require that a special wash be used before you insert the strip for interpretation; when buying a glucose meter, make sure that you have complete instructions on how to use it from the manufacturer's representative and that you know what strips and other equipment are needed.

Of course, self-testing is valuable only if you know how to use the information. Within minutes, you can know whether your blood sugar is too high, too low, or in the normal range. You should feel comfortable with the information and confident of your ability to take whatever corrective measures might be indicated. (Specific guidelines on problem solving are presented in other chapters in this book; your doctor can also tell you how to use self-testing to achieve better diabetes control.)

How to Use Self-Testing

The whole purpose of self-testing is to learn more about your body and how it reacts to various situations as far as levels of blood glucose are concerned and then to use this information to bring your diabetes under better control. Self-Care physicians and diabetes educators repeatedly stress that each patient is different. For example, not everyone has the same lowering of blood glucose from a specific dose of insulin and not everyone has the same effect from eating a specific food. The only way you can know how to anticipate a certain effect is to know how your body normally responds. And this is where self-testing is of particular value.

One of the first things patients in the Diabetes Self-Care Program learn is how to keep an accurate diary and how to use it in future problem solving. To make this easier, a special Self-Care chart, reproduced here, has been developed by Katharine Alling, a diabetes educator and executive director of the Diabetes Control Foundation in Rochester, N.Y. At first it may seem like a lot of unnecessary work to keep such a detailed diary, but most patients find that it takes only a few minutes a day and that it is invaluable in achieving tight blood glucose control. In fact, success for Self-Care patients is denoted by staying in the gray zone, meaning their blood glucose ranges between 50 and 150 mg/dl, the range that is generally recognized as being normal. This range is represented by the shaded area on the Alling chart.

Charting, Step by Step

You should keep a daily diary, which you will find is useful to both you and your doctor. Keep a separate chart for each day—this gives you a running record and also will enable you to spot recurring patterns. For example, women often require more insulin during the week to ten days before menstruation, a pattern that will show up in reviewing diaries kept over several months.

Initially, Self-Care patients are instructed to measure their blood glucose at least six or seven times each day. The after-meal measurements should be an hour after starting a meal; the before-breakfast one should be before injecting insulin (at least a half hour before breakfast). In addition, Self-Care patients take a 3 A.M. blood sugar for the first day or two while learning the program and also to better gauge what happens during the night. Blood glucose tends to be its lowest at about this time; if it is in the hypoglycemic range, insulin dosages will have to be adjusted accordingly.

The results of all blood glucose measurements should be entered on the appropriate lines and also recorded as dots on the graph. The graph entry should be to the nearest quarter hour of the time of testing and to the nearest 5 mg/dl of blood glucose. The dots are connected to form a blood glucose profile, or curve.

Insulin injections also are entered in the section just below the graph. The time of each injection (to the nearest quarter hour) is entered in this section and also is indicated with an upward arrow just below the time bar. Both the number of units and type of insulin should be recorded. (Insulin types are abbreviated as follows on the chart: N for NPH and L for Lente, both intermediate-acting; R for Regular or S for Semilente, both short-acting; and P for Protamine Zinc or U for Ultralente, both long-acting.) The site of injection, for example, left thigh or right bicep, also should be recorded.

Food and drinks (with the exception of water or other noncaloric beverages) should be recorded in the lower portion of the chart. The quota refers to grams of carbohydrates allowed for the meal and snack.

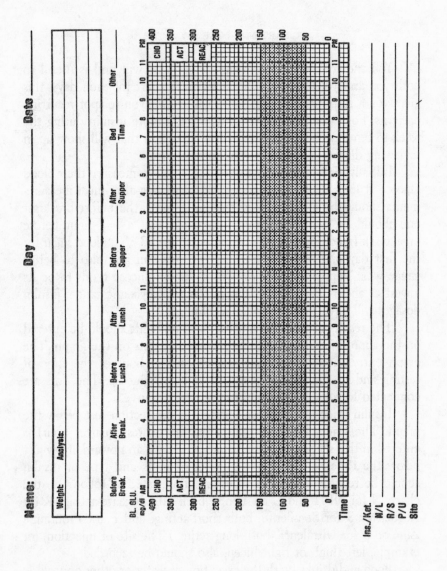

BREAKFAST - SNACKS		Quota:		LUNCH-SNACKS		Quota:		SUPPER-SNACKS		Quota:	
Time:		MEA-SURE	GMS CHO	Time:		MEA-SURE	GMS CHO	Time:		MEA-SURE	CHO

List each item and indicate the total number of grams (if known) and the grams of carbohydrates. To help you see the effect of the carbohydrate intake on your blood glucose curve, their intake also should be recorded at the top of the chart under CHO. Each square represents 10 grams of carbohydrates. Indicate the quota with a downward arrow and the amount actually consumed by filling in the appropriate number of boxes.

Activity (ACT) is recorded just below the CHO section on the chart. Each entry will cover a part of the day: morning, afternoon, and evening. The degree of activity should be graded on a scale of one to five as follows:

1 = minimal activity
   (working at a desk, resting, etc.)
2 = less than usual for the period
3 = average for the period
4 = more than usual for the period
5 = maximal activity

Block out one small box for each gradation; for example, filling in three boxes horizontally will indicate average activity for the period.

The final, and one of the most important, entries deals with insulin reactions, the section labeled REAC, which is beneath ACT in the graph. Entries should be made vertically and recorded to the nearest quarter hour of their onset. They are graded according to their severity on a scale of one to five:

1 = mild signs of impending reaction
2 = obvious symptoms of reaction
3 = moderately severe reaction
4 = severe reaction
5 = maximal reaction experienced

Whenever possible, blood glucose tests should be made to determine the level at which reactions occur and also the levels that mark the different gradations.

At the end of each day, it's a good idea to take a few minutes to analyze or explain unusual circumstances, such as fluctuations in blood glucose or departures from normal activities. For example, if you became angry over an incident in the office shortly before lunch, this might explain why your prelunch glucose was higher than normal. Or if you missed your bus and walked a half mile to work, the extra activity might explain an episode of hypoglycemia.

To better illustrate how the daily diary might be used, the Self-Care Program gives patients sample graphs of typical patients and situations. The model graph of David P. reproduced here is used to instruct Self-Care patients and health professionals in the fine points of charting.

David is five feet, eleven inches tall and usually weighs 167 pounds (76 kg), a weight he maintains on a diet of 2,200 calories per day. He exercises regularly using Nautilus equipment at his health club; he also jogs and plays a weekly game of squash.

The day illustrated on this chart was a Thursday in January. As is true with most people, David's management strategies vary with different days of the week, and noting the day as well as the date is therefore important in analyzing his data. On this morning, he weighed himself and recorded his weight at the top of the chart. His first test revealed a fasting blood glucose of 118 mg/dl at 7 A.M., and he administered his morning insulin at that time: 20 units of NPH (N) and 10 of Regular (R), injecting into his right thigh, site C-8 (see site rotation chart, p. 64–65). He recorded these events on the vertical 7 A.M. line of his graph, both above the time line for the blood glucose and below it for the insulin, and he posted the test result numerically above the graph as well. The numerical record enables David to transmit detail quickly to his physician by phone should need arise, and it facilitates statistical analyses that may be of interest from time to time.

David's daily total of insulin (45 units) is calculated as 0.6 units per kilogram of body weight. It is administered as a combination of NPH and Regular before breakfast; Regular before supper; and NPH before bed. Forty-five minutes after injecting his morning insulin, David ate his usual breakfast, which is low in carbohydrates and high in protein and fat. This is designed to prevent the high blood glucose

Name: DAVID P. _____ **Day** THURSDAY **Date** JAN. 13

| Weight: 167 | Animals: NAUTILUS IN A.M. LUNCH WITH BRADLEY. ATE LESS THAN EXPECTED. MEAN AFTERNOON; GIVEN MONTGOMERY CASE, DI OUT, ETC. REACTION. EXTRA R FOR BOUNCE, AND DELAYED DINNER. CAROL SORE RE LEASE, BUT NICE EVENING. |

BL. GLU.

Before Break.	After Break.	Before Lunch	After Lunch	Before Supper	After Supper	Bed Time	Other
118	142	61	148	236	127	139	114 3:45 P.M. 43

ins./Ket.

®/L	20	7
®/S	10	
P/U	11 (3+)	
Site	R.THIGH 8 L.ARM 4	BELLY 12

BREAKFAST · SNACKS Time: 7:45	MEA-SURE Quota: 15	GMS CHO	LUNCH · SNACKS Time: 12:30	MEA-SURE Quota: 100	GMS CHO	SUPPER · SNACKS Time: 7:15	MEA-SURE Quota: 100	GMS CHO
Boiled Egg	1	.5	Roll	1	5	Rock C.G. Hen	1	30
Toast Buttered	1	14	Antipasto	Sm.	21	Green Beans	1/2 c	11
Coffee, Black	2	–	Linguini w/clam	1/2 c	30	Stuffing	1/2 c	45
Bacon Strips	2	–	Salad	1	5	Sweet Potato	1	5
			Veal Francaise	1	8	Salad	1	2
			Wine	14.5	20	Wine	6oz	8
						Baked Apple	1	20
					89			101
			4:00			11:15		
			Milk	8oz	12	Crackers	4	8
						Cheese	1oz	4

© 1982, Katharine Alling

rise that typically follows breakfast, a meal eaten after an overnight fast and at a time when blood glucose is naturally rising anyway.

The items he ate for breakfast are listed in the diet section of the chart on page 41, and the serving size is indicated as "measure." From these entries, and using a standard carbohydrate guide, David determined the carbohydrate content of his meal in grams. He transferred the total to the top section of the graph (CHO) as follows: starting with the vertical line that represents to the nearest quarter hour the time at which he began his meal, and using one square for each 10 grams of carbohydrates, he graphed his carbohydrates to the nearest 5 grams. The chevron over the end of the bar indicates that he perfectly met his quota, as recorded in the space beside the words "Breakfast–Snacks" in the food columns.

At work, an hour after finishing his breakfast, David tested his blood glucose again and found that it had risen less than 25 mg/dl, to 142 mg/dl. He was scheduled to have lunch that day with an important client and expected it to be a larger meal than he was used to at that hour. He also expected that the encounter would be tense and stressful, so in anticipation of a high rise in blood glucose after lunch, he worked out on the Nautilus machine in his firm's gym during the midmorning. He recorded this strenuous activity on the graph's second bar (ACT), using a graded scale of one to five, where three denotes typical activity for the period in question, and one and five minimal and maximal, respectively. David judged his workout to be deserving of a four since, though it left him feeling well exercised and refreshed, it was not particularly taxing. He left confidently for his luncheon appointment, having found his blood glucose to be 61 mg/ dl before leaving his office.

The luncheon proved to be less stressful than David had feared. It was also less rich in carbohydrates than he had expected, and since his client, who was on a new diet, preferred to forgo dessert, David did too. He therefore met his luncheon's carbohydrate quota of 100 grams. The afternoon went poorly despite the success of the luncheon meeting, and by three-thirty David was feeling terrible. He'd been assigned a case he dreaded, he'd learned that a rental deal he and his wife had hoped to negotiate for the summer had fallen through, and his secretary had left early, her work unfinished, to see her dentist for severe pain. David's head ached, his mouth tasted awful, and he couldn't concentrate. It wasn't until he saw his hand trembling over his work and felt the perspiration spring out on his face and chest that he realized he was having an insulin reaction.

A test result of 43 mg/dl confirmed hypoglycemia, and he quickly drank 8 ounces of milk from a container in the office's small refrigerator. He suspected that the morning's exercise, even though it had not exhausted him, had been too strenuous for his glucose reserves, and that he should probably have had the milk when he returned to the office from lunch. Regarding the reaction as moderately severe but not devastating, he awarded it a three on a scale of one to five, and he recorded the reaction vertically in the third section of the graph (REAC).

As a probable result of a posthypoglycemic bounce, David's blood glucose was up to 236 mg/dl when he arrived home at six o'clock. Because he is somewhat compulsive, he refused to eat dinner until he had regained control. To help this along, he injected 11 units of Regular insulin (3 more than usual). The delay of the dinner she had prepared for him annoyed his wife, Carol, who was upset anyway about the failure of the hoped-for summer lease, and they quarreled during the hour and a half that elapsed before David would confirm that he was now in a position to eat. He indicated the resultant emotional stress with a star in the activity section, but the stress was not sufficient to keep his blood glucose elevated in the face of the increased, fast-acting insulin. By seven-thirty, he and Carol were sitting down to a good dinner, over which they discussed alternative summer plans. They spent a quiet evening together (a two in the activity section), talking and listening to music. Before bed, David administered his final insulin for the day, 7 units of NPH, and had a cheese-and-cracker snack containing 12 grams of carbohydrates.

David's postdinner and bedtime tests were both moderate, and he ended the day feeling that he'd done a fair job of management: he'd been in the normal zone all day, except for a brief excursion following an avoidable insulin reaction. And he'd learned something valuable about the need for food after activity.

His analysis of the day's events, recorded at the top of the page, indicates in abbreviated form what factors he believes influenced his control. Though brief, they will refresh his memory for guidance in planning his management of similar days to come.

While keeping this kind of a careful chart may take a few extra minutes each day, Self-Care patients and doctors alike agree that it is well worth the effort. As noted by Katharine Alling, "Although David's blood glucose dipped down beneath the gray band once in the late afternoon and then bounced too high, in general the day went well despite stress and other difficulties. A moment's study will reveal that a chart less carefully kept would deny us the necessary data for a meaningful analysis of what David had accomplished."

You can begin keeping your own daily chart. You can set up your own or you can order sets of the Alling chart duplicated in this book by contacting the Diabetes Control Foundation, 215 Sandringham Road, Rochester, N.Y. 14610. As noted earlier, these charts not only are helpful to individual patients in learning more about how their bodies respond to a variety of circumstances, they also are very useful for doctors to review periodically. "A good diary allows you to more accurately discuss problems with your doctor," says Dr. Peterson. "Also, as you learn more about yourself and your diabetes, you will find that many things that didn't seem to have an explanation will become more easily understood when you look at them in terms of your diary and the various circumstances involved. By measuring what you are doing and keeping good records, you will soon become both the expert and the master of your diabetes."

5

The Importance of Insulin
in Controlling Diabetes

The treatment of diabetes has a long and somewhat checkered history. Insulin—the essential substance in controlling the kind of diabetes in which the pancreas has ceased to produce the hormone—was not discovered until 1921, meaning that for type 1 diabetics there was no truly effective treatment before that date. Most patients with this form of the disease died within a few years, often after being subjected to a variety of rigorous diets. For centuries doctors have known that food has a dramatic effect on the disease. Very often the treatment advocated was to withhold food to the point of starvation. Other patients were subjected to a variety of fad diets, most with little or no scientific basis. As noted by Joan Choppin, a dietitian with the Diabetes Self-Care Program, "Some patients were helped by these diets, others were not, and some were even made worse. There are tales of patients being forced to drink their own sweetened urine, or of being fed large amounts of candy daily to replace lost sugar."

But every now and then these early physicians serendipitously stumbled onto valid concepts. In 1796, for example, Dr. John Rollo, a surgeon general in the British Royal Artillery, advocated a diet high in animal foods: in essence, a diet high in fat and protein and low in carbohydrates. Although this was before foods were classified according to their individual nutrients, Dr. Rollo had identified foods now known to be high in carbohydrates as factors in diabetes. Because of this, he is credited with devising the first effective means of treating diabetes. Today, calculating carbohydrates and balancing them with the proper amount of insulin is a major factor in the self-care of diabetes.

In 1913, Dr. Frederick M. Allen of the Rockefeller Institute for Medical Research, since renamed Rockefeller University, devised a diet high in fiber and low in calories. While Dr. Allen's diet provided a good deal of bulk with little in the way of nutrients, it is a forerunner to today's high-fiber diet, another valid dietary concept in treating diabetes.

Although diet is important in treating type 1 diabetics, it cannot serve as the sole treatment. A rigorous diet low in calories and carbohydrates may prolong the life of a diabetic patient, but without the vital hormone, the person will eventually die of the disease. Thus, it was not until 1921 and the discovery of insulin by Drs. Frederick Banting and Charles Best that people with type 1 diabetes had any hope of long-term survival.

The story of how Drs. Banting and Best discovered insulin is a fascinating one, involving two young men with no previous research experience and very little in the way of laboratory facilities or support. Frederick Banting was a twenty-nine-year-old orthopedic surgeon at the University of Western Ontario, and Charles Best was a recent graduate in physiology and biochemistry from the University of Toronto. As a young veteran of World War I just embarking on a medical career, Dr. Banting found he had few patients to occupy his time and mind. He spent long hours in the university library, reading papers on a wide range of medical topics. He ran across one by Dr. Moses Barron of the University of Minnesota, in which the author speculated that an as yet unknown substance secreted by the pancreas might be of value in treating diabetes mellitus.

Dr. Banting, who was preparing a paper on the function of the pancreas at the time, made a note to himself to set up an experiment with dogs in which he would attempt to isolate this substance. He discussed his idea with several of his London, Ontario, colleagues, who encouraged him to pursue it further. But since the research facilities at Western Ontario were minimal, he took his research proposal to an authority in carbohydrate metabolism, Dr. John J. R. Macleod, at the University of Toronto. Dr. Macleod, a Scot of the old European school, was doubtful, but finally agreed to let Dr. Banting use a laboratory and some research animals for the summer of 1921. Dr. Macleod also enlisted one of his students, twenty-two-year-old Charles Best, to work with Dr. Banting as an unpaid research assistant.

The rest of the story is history. After long, often frustrating hours in the sweltering attic laboratory, the two finally produced the results they were seeking in the early morning hours of July 31, 1921. They had succeeded in extracting a small amount of substance from a dog pancreas and injected it in another animal whose pancreas had been removed. Within a short time, there was no longer any sugar in the dog's urine, and the animal's high level of blood glucose fell by half. Over the next few weeks they successfully repeated the experiment on other diabetic dogs with similar results—the pancreatic extract lowered the blood glucose and cleared the urine of sugar.

Later that year, their discovery was announced to the medical community and was picked up by newspapers around the world. Desperate diabetics began clamoring for the miracle substance, which the researchers first named "isletin" for the islets of Langerhans, and then switched to the more easily pronounced "insulin." But several problems had to be overcome before patients were to receive insulin. For one thing, it had never been tried on a human being. The researchers remedied this by injecting it first in themselves to make sure that it was safe, and then administered it in January 1922 to a thirteen-year-old boy, Leonard Thompson, who was near death from diabetes in a Toronto hospital. The effect on Thompson was nothing short of miraculous. He was a tiny, listless child whose growth was severely retarded—he weighed barely 64 pounds. Five months after receiving his first series of insulin injections, which lowered his blood sugar from 470 mg/dl to a normal range, Thompson was discharged from the hospital.

The short-term therapy had not cured his diabetes, however; by October 1923, he was back in the hospital, weighing just 60 pounds in severe diabetic ketoacidosis. He was then put on a daily schedule of four insulin injections and was given a diet high in fat (160 grams), a moderate amount of protein (50 grams), and relatively low in carbohydrates (100 grams). Over the next few weeks and months, his condition improved, and he began to grow and to recover normal bodily functions. He was able to engage in normal boyhood pursuits, including playing baseball. He lived another thirteen years with insulin therapy, dying in 1935 of bronchopneumonia and complications of diabetes.

In those early years, many problems remained to be solved before insulin became widely available. Over the next few years, Dr. Best developed techniques to extract the insulin from pork and beef pancreases, and drug companies in Canada, the United States, and elsewhere began producing it in adequate amounts to treat diabetics around the world. The drug was in such demand and considered so important that the League of Nations oversaw its distribution. Millions of people with diabetes throughout the world owe a lasting debt to Drs. Banting and Best for their pioneering research. The 1923 Nobel Prize in medicine and physiology was awarded to Drs. Banting and Macleod. Honoring Dr. Macleod instead of Dr. Best has been a continuing source of controversy; at the time, Dr. Banting insisted that his part of the prize be shared with Dr. Best, and in the ensuing years both men received many honors throughout the world. Dr. Banting died of injuries suffered in a plane crash during World War II; Dr. Best devoted the rest of his career to diabetes research, which is continuing today at the Banting and Best Department of Medical Research in Toronto.

Although the discovery of insulin was a giant step in the treatment of diabetes, it is not a cure for the disease. It controls the diabetes, making it possible to lead a reasonably normal, productive life. This is why the crux of bringing diabetes under control, particularly the type 1 form of the disease, in which the pancreas produces little or no insulin, centers on understanding and managing insulin injections. Insulin is a protein hormone that is destroyed by the digestive process; therefore, it must be administered directly into the bloodstream instead of being taken by mouth in pill form. The most common method of administering insulin is by subcutaneous injection, although a growing number of patients are using insulin pumps. These are portable, computerized devices that are designed to mimic the natural pancreas by administering varying amounts of insulin through an indwelling needle and catheter. (Other methods of administering insulin, for example, by inhalation or in an oral form, are under study, but are not available at this time.)

Regardless of the method of administration, the goal of insulin therapy is to maintain the amount of glucose circulating in the blood at levels as near normal as possible. In the early days of insulin therapy, this was achieved with four injections a day. As more types of insulin were developed, this strategy changed. Some insulins go to work and reach their peak effectiveness fairly quickly; others are slower-acting. By combining the fast- and slow-acting insulins, doctors were able to reduce the number of injections required. In fact, many patients were switched to regimens that required only one injection of a slow- or intermediate-acting insulin a day. Patients were taught to test their urine daily to make sure that it did not contain sugar. They also were put on a rigid eating schedule designed to match the peaks of insulin effectiveness with the intake of food.

In the last decade, this approach to managing diabetes has been reevaluated, and many experts, including doctors at the Diabetes Self-Care Program, now feel that for most diabetics, the once-a-day injection cannot effectively control the disease. More accurate methods of assessing overall control of blood glucose have proved this to be the case. Instead of maintaining blood glucose within a normal range, it may swing from too high to too low several times during a twenty-four-hour period. Thus the insulin system advocated in the Diabetes Self-Care Program calls for multiple insulin injections each day, with careful self-monitoring to make the necessary dosage adjustments. There are several advantages to this approach. It comes closer to mimicking normal pancreatic function than a single daily injection. It also allows the person with diabetes more freedom in timing food intake, exercising, and engaging in other normal day-to-day activities. As Drs. Peterson and Jovanovic repeatedly remind their patients in the Diabetes Self-Care Program, "The trick is to match your insulin peaks with the peaks of blood glucose." Since most people eat three meals a day, this means planning for three insulin peaks—something that is almost impossible to accomplish with a single daily injection. "On the other hand," Dr. Jovanovic notes, "if you are not going to eat, then you need only your basal insulin and not the usual three injections."

KNOW YOUR INSULIN

Today's diabetic patient must understand the different kinds of insulins and how to match their peak effectiveness with the times of greatest insulin demand; namely, following a meal that contains carbohydrates and, to a lesser degree, protein, or during periods of stress or other circumstances that increase the need for insulin. Since different insulins vary in onset, peak, and duration of action, one of the first things a person with diabetes should know is the type of insulin he or she uses. (The following table gives the approximate data for each type.) Most diabetic patients take two different kinds of insulin: Regular, or fast-acting insulin and an intermediate- or slow-acting one.

Regular insulin begins acting within thirty to sixty minutes, peaks in two to four hours, and has a total duration of action of four to six hours. Thus, if you take only Regular insulin, you need an injection every four to six hours. In contrast, an intermediate-acting insulin such as NPH or Lente begins acting in three to four hours, peaks in eight to twelve hours, and lasts for eighteen hours. This type of insulin provides for a slow, steady regulation of blood glucose, but may not be adequate to handle the sharp rises that follow a meal containing carbohydrates or situations that call for extra insulin. The regimen favored at the Diabetes Self-Care Program combines Regular and NPH insulin, divided into three injections. This regimen results in about four insulin peaks per day and covers three meals, several snacks, and the early-morning (dawn phenomenon) period of insulin resistance experienced by many people with diabetes.

TABLE

CHARACTERISTICS OF DIFFERENT INSULINS

Insulin	Characteristic	Onset of Action (hrs)	Peak Action (hrs)	Total Duration (hrs)
Regular	Fast-acting	.5–1	2–4	4–6
Semilente	Fast-acting	1–2	3–6	4–6
NPH	Intermediate-acting	3–4	8–12	18
Lente	Intermediate-acting	3–4	10–16	20–24
Ultralente	Long-acting	4–6	14–20	32+
PZI	Long-acting	6–8	14–20	32+

Many factors must be taken into consideration in arriving at an ideal insulin dosage. Even then, many variables can intervene to alter insulin needs. This is why many diabetic patients will be hospitalized initially until a suitable regimen can be worked out to meet individual or special needs; nevertheless, they may have to adjust their dosage to cover different circumstances. For example, women of childbearing age may need considerably more insulin in the week before their menstrual period. A cold or other infection may sharply increase the need for insulin. An emotional upset often sends blood sugar soaring and increases insulin demand. Conversely, vigorous exercise decreases insulin need. (Common factors affecting insulin requirements are listed in the following table.) The dosage formulas outlined here are used by the Diabetes Self-Care Program to arrive at a general dosage; further adjustments are then made according to individual responses and needs. "It's important to remember that each person is different," cautions Dr. Jovanovic. "What works for one patient will not necessarily work for another, even though they appear to be very similar."

One of the first factors to be considered in calculating insulin dosages is total body weight in kilograms. To find your approximate weight in kilograms, divide the number of pounds you weigh by 2.2. Thus a person who tips the scale at 132 pounds weighs 60 kilograms.

This gives you the first figure that doctors use in calculating a total insulin dosage. Most normal adults who are moderately active require 0.6 units of insulin per kilogram over a twenty-four-hour period. Thus, if the 60-kilogram patient falls into this average range, the total daily insulin dosage would be 36 units. Since a number of factors influence insulin requirement, the ratio may have to be altered accordingly. The general ratios used at the Diabetes Self-Care Program are:

Patient	Insulin requirement
Athlete (e.g., marathon runner)	0.5 units/kg/24 hours
Normal active adult	0.6 units/kg/24 hours
Premenstrual woman or person with an infection	0.7 units/kg/24 hours
Pregnant woman	0.6–1 units/kg/24 hours depending on week of pregnancy
Adolescent during growth spurt or any patient during episode of acidosis	2 units/kg/24 hours

Using this table, a normally active 60-kilogram adult who is not premenstrual or has no infection or other problem that increases the need for insulin will require about 36 units of insulin during a typical twenty-four-hour period. This will be divided into two or three injections, and adjustments may be made based on blood sugar measurements, food intake, exercise, and other factors affecting insulin or blood sugar. As emphasized before, patients should not adjust their dosages themselves until they are experienced in solving insulin problems and calculating dosages.

The rationale for combining insulins is fairly simple: Regular is given to cover meals and an intermediate- or slow-acting insulin, such as NPH, is used to cover the basal metabolism as well as some food. In other words, if a person with diabetes is not going to eat for a given period of time, little or no Regular insulin will be required; the NPH or other long-acting insulin will cover metabolic needs during the fasting period. Thus, the next step in establishing an insulin regimen is calculating how much food should be consumed in a typical day and then matching it with the right amount of insulin. To do this, you must learn how to count calories and also how to distribute them among carbohydrates, protein, and fat. While this sounds complicated, most people quickly master the art of counting calories and calculating carbohydrates and other nutrients in a few days. With a little practice, you too will be able to do this simply by looking at a serving on a plate. (For more details, see Chapter 6.)

To better understand how to match insulin and food intake, let's go back to the hypothetical patient described earlier. You will recall that this patient weighs 132 pounds, or 60 kilograms, and is a moderately active adult. Let's assume that the 60 kilograms is an ideal weight for this person and that the activity level also is about right. Using the following table, we can determine the total number of calories that should be consumed in a typical day:

Weight Status	Calories Needed per Kilogram for Activity Level		
	Sedentary	Moderately Active	Very Active
Overweight	12–20	25	35
Normal weight	25	30	40
Underweight	30	35	45

Using this table, we can see that our normal-weight 60-kilogram patient should eat about 30 calories per kilogram to maintain his or her present weight and activity level. Multiplying 60 by 30, we arrive at 1,800 calories per day. The Self-Help Program recommends that 40 percent of these calories come from carbohydrates, 20 to 25 percent from protein, and 35 to 40 percent from fat. The next step is to calculate the number of grams of carbohydrates, protein, and fat that should be consumed each day. Each gram of carbohydrate and protein contains 4 calories; there are 9 calories per gram of fat. Thus the following formula, again based on meeting the energy needs of a 60-kilogram moderately active person, can be used to calculate the specific number of grams in each nutrient group:

40% of 1,800 = 720 calories of carbohydrates
÷ 4 = 180 grams of carbohydrates

20–25% of 1,800 = 360–450 calories of protein
÷ 4 = 90–112 grams of protein

35–40% of 1,800 = 630–720 calories of fat
÷ 9 = 70–80 grams of fat

Since carbohydrates are the most important dietary variable affecting insulin needs, their distribution through the day is a critical factor in matching insulin and food. Ideally, the insulin schedule should be matched to a person's eating schedule and also to the amount and types of foods consumed in each meal. In general, one unit of Regular insulin covers 8 to 10 grams of carbohydrates. For example, the normal insulin requirement for our 60-kilogram moderately active diabetic patient would be 36 units a day. Since this person has a total carbohydrate allowance of about 180 grams and 90 to 112 grams of protein, the 36 units should be adequate to cover basal needs and the glucose produced by this food, provided the person engages in a moderate amount of physical activity. Although more than half of the protein consumed also is converted to glucose, the effect on blood sugar is slower and not as critical as the effect of a carbohydrate meal, especially one that contains simple sugars.

Since the effect of carbohydrates on blood sugar begins fifteen to thirty minutes after you begin eating, insulin is administered to achieve its peak effectiveness when blood glucose rises after a meal containing carbohydrates. Therefore, the typical multiple-dose regimen combining Regular and NPH insulin would call for an injection of NPH and Regular insulin before breakfast to cover the carbohydrates consumed at breakfast and also to counter the increased insulin resistance experienced by many people during the early morning hours, the so-called dawn phenomenon. By lunchtime, there should be enough insulin from the NPH, which begins to act in three to four hours, plus some remaining from the morning Regular, to cover this meal, provided it contains the allotted amount of carbohydrates. Since most people eat the largest meal of the day in the evening, it follows that a strong peak of insulin will be required after dinner. Typically, this is covered by an injection of Regular insulin taken before dinner. To maintain normal blood sugar through the night, an additional injection of NPH must be administered before going to bed.

To calculate how much of each kind of insulin should be given in each injection, the following formula is used:

One sixth of the total dose is given as NPH before going to bed, or 1/6 of 36 = 6 units of NPH before bed.

One sixth of the total dose is given as Regular before dinner, or 1/6 of 36 = 6 units of Regular before dinner.

Remaining two thirds is given in a 2:1 ratio of NPH:Regular before breakfast, or 2/3 of 24 = 16 units of NPH and 1/3 of 24 = 8 units of Regular before breakfast.

How to Take Insulin

One of the first things a person with diabetes must learn is how to inject insulin. At first, many people are reluctant to inject themselves. They may associate injections with childhood fears of getting shots when they visited a pediatrician. Others may be reluctant to inject themselves, especially in public places, because of fears they will be associated with drug addicts. Both fears are groundless; when properly administered with the proper syringe, the injections involve little or no pain. As for the fear of being mistaken for an addict, simply explaining that you have diabetes and must take injections regularly to lead a normal life should suffice. But it is also a good idea to carry a statement from a doctor verifying that the needles and medication are for diabetes, and, of course, all diabetic patients should wear a Medic Alert bracelet or identifying symbol. What's more, most diabetic patients learn ways of injecting themselves, even in public places like restaurants, that are barely noticeable to others, including people at the same table. (Dr. Jovanovic teaches her patients how to inject

themselves under the table in a restaurant in such a manner that not
even dining companions know what is going on.)

All newly diagnosed diabetic patients who require insulin should
be taught to inject themselves by a physician or other trained diabetes
educator. Even so, it is useful for patients to periodically review their
technique to make sure they are following the correct procedure.

At present, insulin comes in two concentrations: U-40 and
U-100. The U stands for units, and the 40 and 100 indicate the
strength. Until recently there was also a U-80; this has been removed
from the market and eventually there will only be one strength of
insulin, U-100, to avoid confusion between the two strengths. The
insulin syringes are color-coded: red is for U-40 and orange or black is
for U-100. Before filling a syringe (drawing insulin), make sure that
you are using the proper one for your insulin.

Before beginning, assemble all the supplies you need: syringe,
alcohol swabs, and insulin bottle(s). Check the expiration date on the
bottle and also make sure that the top has not been damaged. To
minimize the hazard of infection, wash hands thoroughly with soap
and water.

To mix the insulin, gently roll the bottle between your hands.
Avoid shaking it because this may cause air bubbles to form. Clean the
top of the bottle with an alcohol swab.

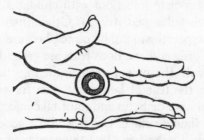

*Gently roll insulin bottle to mix: do not
shake.*

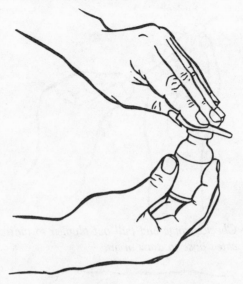

Clean bottle top with alcohol swab.

Check your syringe to make sure that you have the proper type. If you are mixing two types of insulin, you can use the same syringe, but be sure to put in the Regular insulin first. (It is easy to distinguish Regular insulin from NPH and other intermediate- or slow-acting insulins because Regular is clear and the others have a cloudy appearance.) Draw air into the syringe by pulling the plunger to the indicated dose. For example, if you are drawing 9 units of Regular, pull the plunger to 9 units and then inject the air into the bottle of insulin by inserting the needle into the rubber stopper on the top of the bottle and pushing in the plunger. Turn the bottle and syringe upside down and slowly pull the plunger down about 5 units past your dose. Inspect the syringe for air bubbles; if there are none, push the top of the plunger to the line that marks your exact dose and remove it from the bottle. If there are bubbles, gently tap the syringe with your finger where the bubbles appear until they disappear; then remove syringe.

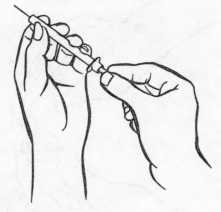

*Check syringe and pull out plunger to indi-
cated dose to draw in air.*

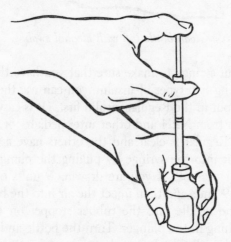

*Inject air into insulin bottle by inserting nee-
dle into top and pushing plunger down.*

If you are mixing insulins, roll each bottle and clean the tops as
just described. If you are taking 12 units of NPH and 6 units of
Regular, to follow the example for our hypothetical patient, start by
drawing 12 units of air into the syringe and injecting this into the
NPH bottle. Remove the syringe, and fill it with 6 units of air, which

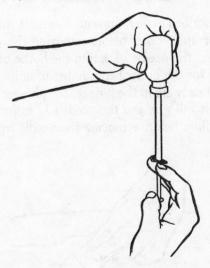

Turn bottle upside down and slowly pull plunger down about 5 units beyond dose.

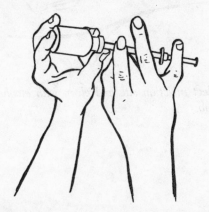

Check syringe for air bubbles; if bubbles have formed, gently flick syringe until they move to top. Push plunger to exact dose and remove needle from bottle.

you will then inject into the bottle of Regular insulin. But instead of withdrawing the syringe, turn the bottle upside down and, following the procedure described earlier, draw up 6 units of Regular insulin. Be sure to check for air bubbles before removing the needle from the bottle. Next, insert the needle back into the bottle of NPH and draw back the plunger for the prescribed number of units. Since 6 units of Regular insulin already are in the syringe, the plunger should be pulled back to 18, which will give you the needed 12 units of NPH. Again, check for air bubbles before removing the needle from the bottle.

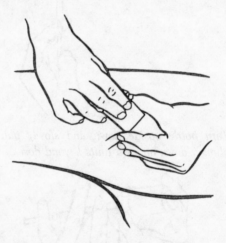

Select injection site and clean with alcohol swab.

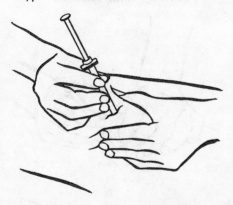

Pinch up a fold of skin and underlying fatty tissue (about one to two inches). Inject needle at a forty-five- to ninety-degree angle.

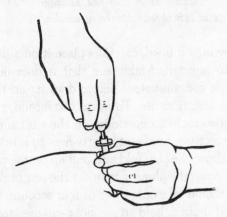

Pull plunger up 2 to 4 units and then inject remaining insulin by pressing plunger in.

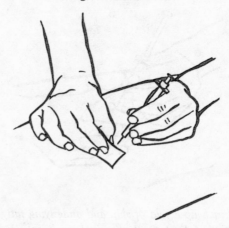

*Remove needle and wipe injection site gently
with alcohol swab. Do not massage or rub
site as this speeds uptake of insulin.*

After the syringe is filled, carefully place it on a flat surface until you are ready to inject it. Make sure that it does not touch other objects or become contaminated. Before drawing up the insulin, you should select the injection site. To inject the insulin, pinch up a fold of skin (one to two inches, depending on the site) and with a single quick motion, inject the needle at a forty-five- to ninety-degree angle into the skin. Release the skin fold and pull up on the plunger about 2 to 4 units. Push down the plunger to inject the rest of the insulin. The entire injection should take only three or four seconds. Gently remove the needle and, if desired, hold an alcohol swab over the site for a few seconds. Ordinarily, the injection site should not be rubbed or massaged since this may affect the amount of time it takes the insulin to enter the circulation. But if you want to eat soon or speed the insulin action, you can do so by gently rubbing the area with a warm washcloth.

To prevent possible injury to others or abuse of the syringe, you should replace the needle shield and bend it back and forth until the needle breaks before you discard the syringe. Be careful where you discard used needles and other items, such as the lancets used in testing blood glucose. Someone emptying a wastebasket containing these items, for example, may cut himself or herself and risk getting hepatitis or other infections transmitted by blood contact.

Insulin should be injected into the subcutaneous tissue, the fatty area that lies under the skin and over the muscle. When properly injected into this subcutaneous tissue, the insulin will be absorbed into the bloodstream at a steady rate. There are a number of injection sites, most notably the front and sides of the thighs, the upper outer area of the arms, the buttocks, the abdomen (avoid the waistline and area surrounding the navel, however), and the area above the waistline. The injection sites should be rotated to avoid repeated injections in the same area over a short period of time. This helps avoid hardening or atrophy of the fatty tissue and also avoids the pain and other problems that may be encountered in repeated use of an injection site. Most people develop their own rotation pattern. The following body maps show the various injection sites. Sites may be rotated from left to right sides, front to back, or any other pattern that is convenient. If a lump, shallow depression, or pain develops in a site, avoid using it for a time. A hardening of the fatty tissue can decrease insulin absorption or make injections difficult to administer.

Many people are hesitant to inject insulin in public; for example, at work or when dining out with friends in a restaurant. Dr. Jovanovic urges her patients to prepare the syringe of insulin in advance and then to quietly administer the injection at a site on the upper leg under the table. Some physicians may frown on this practice because it often means injecting through clothing, but Dr. Jovanovic says she has repeatedly done this herself and has never had a problem injecting through clothing or encountered a subsequent infection. Alternatively, you may prefer to excuse yourself and administer the injection in a restroom.

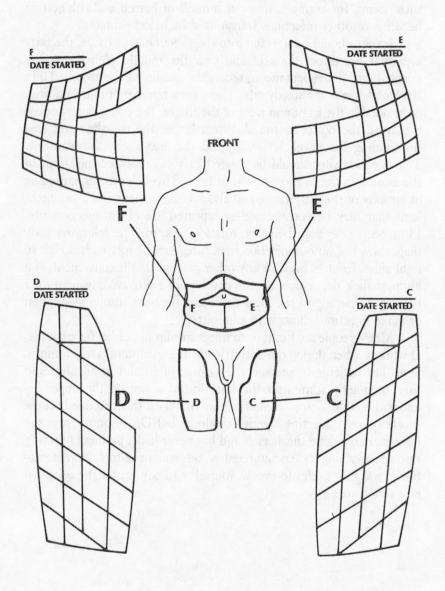

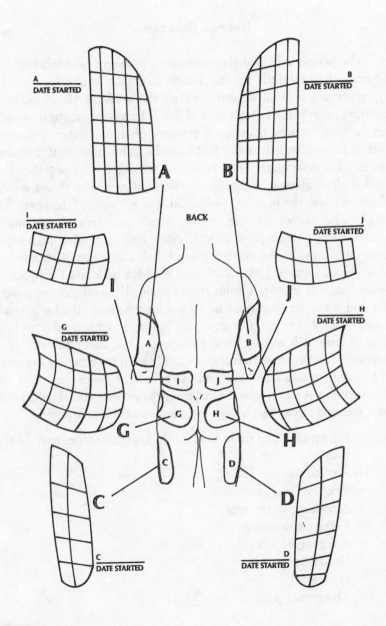

INSULIN REACTIONS

The person with diabetes encounters problems both when there is too much or too little insulin. Taking too much insulin may lead to hypoglycemia, a rapid depletion of all the available blood glucose, resulting in an insulin reaction or shock. The low blood sugar usually can be countered by consuming a source of simple sugar: a glass of milk is recommended in the Self-Care Program because it contains lactose, a simple sugar that is quickly absorbed and provides the needed blood glucose, and protein, which will provide a slower source of glucose over the next few hours. (Milk is not advised, however, for people who cannot tolerate lactose, a common trait among many black adults.) Orange juice, candy, honey, fruit, and other high-sugar foods also provide the needed glucose but may cause a bounce, in which blood sugar will rise rapidly and then fall back into the hypoglycemic range as leftover insulin strikes again. If blood glucose is very low and there are symptoms of an insulin reaction, drinking a small amount (say 4 ounces) of orange juice followed in a few minutes by a glass of milk will quickly raise the glucose but lower the risk of a bounce. Most people with diabetes quickly learn to recognize the signs of an insulin reaction and take steps to counter it. Since the symptoms of an insulin reaction vary from person to person, you should know your warning signs, which may include any of the following:

- A tingling sensation in the mouth, fingers, or other parts of the body
- A cold, clammy feeling
- Paleness
- A buzzing in the ears
- Excessive sweating
- A feeling of weakness or faintness
- Headache
- Hunger
- Abdominal pain

- Irritability and change in mood or personality
- Impaired vision
- Rapid heartbeat and trembling
- Sudden drowsiness
- Sudden awakening from sleep, especially if it is accompanied by other symptoms

If ignored, the reaction may progress to a coma. An insulin reaction sometimes occurs at night when the person is sleeping; inability to waken a person with diabetes is always a sign to call a doctor and to administer a fast source of sugar. This may be an injection of glucagon, which the body almost immediately converts to glucose, or honey or a sugar syrup placed under the tongue, where it will be quickly absorbed into the circulation.

At one time or another, most diabetic patients, including those in good control, will experience an episode of low blood sugar. Possible causes range from taking too much insulin, not eating enough food, engaging in an unusual amount of exercise, or delaying a meal. The initial instinct is to quickly eat something, but in most cases there is time for a reasoned response that will overcome the low blood sugar but not send the blood glucose too high. To make this reasoned response, a diabetic patient should be prepared to cope with the situation before encountering it. This is why doctors advise their patients with diabetes to always carry with them the equipment needed to measure their blood sugar as well as a source of quickly absorbed sugar, such as candy, sugar cubes, fruit, or other sources of simple carbohydrates. Patients in the Diabetes Self-Care Program are advised to experiment with certain readily available foods to determine in advance just how much and how fast they can be expected to increase blood sugar. To do this, measure your blood sugar at a time when you expect that it will be less than 120 mg/dl. If it is below that range, consume a source of sugar; for example, a glass of milk or an apple. Wait fifteen to thirty minutes and measure your blood sugar again. Keep track of the results, and over a period of several days or weeks, experiment with several different foods. Armed with this information, you will be able to gauge what you should take to produce a specific increase in blood glucose.

Although hypoglycemia is a potentially serious event and its warning signs should never be ignored, it is not a cause for panic. In fact, panic or fear may further provoke the situation and prevent you from taking the calm, clear-headed action needed to counteract the reaction. If the insulin reaction has not affected your coordination, it's a good idea to measure your blood glucose to see just how hypoglycemic you are. This takes only a couple of minutes, and will tell you how much and what kind of food you should consume. If it is very low, say in the range of 40 or 50 mg/dl, a fast source of simple sugar is called for. Half a glass of orange juice (4 ounces) should raise blood sugar about 100 mg/dl within a half hour, although this varies from person to person. Eating an apple, a piece of candy, fruit, or other sources of simple sugar will produce similar increases. To prevent bouncing from low to high and back down again, combine the simple sugar with a complex carbohydrate and protein. For example, if the blood sugar is below 70, the Diabetes Self-Care doctors advise drinking a glass of milk and rechecking the blood glucose in fifteen minutes. If it is still low, drink another glass of milk. If this still doesn't work, drink a third glass of milk and eat a slice of bread. Dr. Peterson stresses that the latter is hardly ever necessary.

Of course, low blood sugar is not the only extreme that is potentially hazardous to the diabetic person; high blood sugar also can be life-threatening. The high blood sugar may be caused by not taking enough insulin or failure to absorb insulin that is taken; infection, fever, or other illness; pregnancy; emotional stress; or consumption of more carbohydrates than can be covered by the insulin dosage. The onset of hyperglycemia is slower than that of hypoglycemia, and the early warning signs may go unnoticed, especially if the problem is related to stress or illness. Warning signs include:

- Increased thirst and urination
- Loss of appetite
- Nausea and vomiting
- Weakness

- Large amounts of ketones in the urine
- Blood sugar measurement of more than 300 mg/dl
- Breath will smell fruity (from acetones)
- Dehydration (dry mouth, skin, etc.)
- Fixed, dilated pupils, difficulty in focusing
- Heavy, labored breathing
- Loss of consciousness (diabetic coma)

Regular self-monitoring of blood sugar and adjusting insulin dosages accordingly should be sufficient to avoid ketoacidosis—the serious imbalance in blood chemistry that results when the diabetic starts burning too much body fat because the body is unable to use glucose. When blood sugar reaches a certain level, it is a sign that steps should be taken to lower it. Depending on the circumstances and the level of blood sugar, these may range from skipping a meal to increasing your insulin dosage. In general, a unit of insulin will lower blood glucose by 20 to 60 mg/dl, depending on how high it is, the cause of the hyperglycemia, and individual response to insulin. Again, the best way to counter hyperglycemia is to experiment in advance so you can anticipate how much a unit of insulin will lower your blood glucose.

Test your urine periodically for the presence of ketones. If ketoacidosis does occur, consult a doctor immediately. Since serious dehydration and imbalances in body chemistry, particularly electrolytes, are common features of diabetic ketoacidosis, intravenous administration of fluids is usually required. Insulin also may be administered intravenously or in frequent injections. Other emergency treatment may be required, depending on the severity of the acidosis and the extent of chemical imbalance. In any event, careful monitoring over a period of several days usually is required.

SPECIAL PROBLEMS AND CONSIDERATIONS

As emphasized earlier, each person differs in his or her response to insulin and other factors associated with diabetes. Within a relatively short time—ranging from a few days to several weeks—most people with type 1 diabetes can be brought under control and taught an insulin regimen, reinforced by self-monitoring of blood glucose, that will fit their individual lifestyles. Only a small minority encounter problems such as marked insulin resistance or insulin allergy. Still, diabetic patients should be aware of these potential problems, even though it is unlikely that they will ever experience them.

True insulin allergy is very rare, occurring in only 0.1 percent or one out of every one thousand persons with diabetes. A systemic allergic reaction to insulin should not be confused with the occasional local reaction that might occur at specific injection sites. Insulin allergy is characterized by an almost immediate local reaction that gradually spreads until a wide area is covered with hives or an itching rash. Edema (swelling) may occur, and in rare instances, anaphylactic shock similar to that associated with severe penicillin allergy has been reported.

Sometimes switching to a different kind of insulin (for example, pork instead of beef) may solve the problem, but this is unusual and not always desirable because the offending insulin may have to be used at some future date. The new human insulins also may be tried, but they may not be available. Desensitization is the preferred treatment for insulin allergy. This involves administering very small but gradually increasing doses of insulin over a short period of time, using a mixed solution of both beef and pork insulin. This is done under close medical supervision. If the patient can tolerate lowered doses of insulin without having blood sugar rise dangerously, the desensitization shots may be given every two hours; otherwise they may be given every thirty minutes or hour until desensitization is achieved. Manufacturers of insulin provide desensitization kits that health professionals can use in treating allergic reactions.

Insulin resistance in varying degrees is encountered more frequently than insulin allergies. As the term implies, insulin resistance is characterized by the body's inability to use insulin even though it is available in adequate or even greater than normal quantities. Type 2 diabetic patients are often referred to as insulin-resistant because their pancreases are producing what should be sufficient amounts of the hormone. A number of circumstances can increase insulin resistance in both type 1 and type 2 diabetes, including obesity, infection, pregnancy, and certain drugs, particularly steroids. Many people with type 1 diabetes have periods of insulin resistance that are not related to any identifiable causes. In most of these people, the resistance is due to an increase in insulin-binding immune gamma globulin (IgG) antibodies. Everyone produces a certain amount of these antibodies; for unexplained reasons, a small number of patients will suddenly produce very high quantities. Since insulin binds to the antibodies, very large amounts may be required to ensure that enough will circulate in the body. This type of resistance tends to come and go; the antibodies may reach a very high level and then return to normal without any apparent explanation.

Certain diseases, such as acromegaly (a disorder caused by a pituitary gland tumor that causes excessive secretion of growth hormone) or hemochromatosis (a disorder of iron metabolism that affects the liver and carbohydrate metabolism), may cause insulin resistance. Cirrhosis and other liver diseases also may increase the need for insulin.

Loss or deterioration of the fatty tissue that lies under the skin is still another cause of insulin resistance. This is usually a localized condition caused by overuse of an injection site; the fatty tissue will either atrophy or become hardened. There are also some people who have widespread loss of fatty (adipose) tissue, a disorder called lipodystrophy or lipoatrophy. This may affect a part of the body, such as the upper half or the lower extremities, or it may involve the entire body. This type of lipodystrophy is not the same as the localized atrophy from insulin injections. It is a rare disease that usually occurs in people with type 2 diabetes and certain liver or metabolic disorders.

Traditionally, insulin resistance is defined as the need for more than 200 units of insulin per day for two or more days. According to Dr. Peterson, a more precise and useful definition is the continuing need for more than 2 units of insulin per kilogram per twenty-four hours. Treatment varies according to the cause of the resistance. In cases that are secondary to other diseases, such as infection, treating the underlying cause will often return the insulin need to normal. Insulin resistance due to increased IgG antibodies sometimes can be overcome by using a modified type of insulin that the antibodies are not as likely to recognize and bind to. Very large doses of insulin may be administered, but this requires careful monitoring because the IgG levels may return to normal relatively quickly. In any event, marked insulin resistance requires close monitoring by a doctor.

SUMMING UP

The discovery of insulin in 1921 has enabled millions of people with type 1 diabetes to lead reasonably normal, productive lives. The administration of insulin, however, is not a cure for the disease. The person with diabetes must be constantly attuned to his or her body and must understand the relationship between food and insulin, as well as the many factors that affect the body's need for and use of insulin. Fortunately, today's diabetic patient has many tools that make this task easier than in the past. Foremost among these is the self-monitoring of blood glucose levels. Within minutes, the diabetic can accurately determine the level of blood sugar and take appropriate corrective steps if it is too high or too low. Self-monitoring also makes it possible for the person with diabetes to lead a more flexible life than in the past and still maintain the tight control that most doctors now believe is important not only in helping the diabetic patient feel better but also in possibly preventing some of the long-term complications of the disease.

6

The Importance of Diet

Many people with type 1 diabetes find they are preoccupied with food. This preoccupation is understandable and becomes evident as one listens to a group of patients at a Diabetes Self-Care session. Alice confesses she has recurring dreams about ice cream, and now and then succumbs to the temptation, with the predictable result of sending her blood sugar soaring. Bob tries to analyze what he calls his food rebellions. Rita says she's hungry most of the time, but is trying to lose fifteen pounds. For these patients and the nearly two million other Americans with type 1 diabetes, the Self-Care Program has developed an approach to diet and meal planning that offers considerable flexibility and freedom in selecting foods. In the words of Dr. Peterson, "We like to emphasize that there are no 'bad' or 'off-limits' foods. While some foods obviously have greater health benefits than others, we stress that with proper planning, the type 1 diabetic can eat any and all foods."

This does not mean that Alice can fulfill her dream of bingeing on ice cream or that Rita can head for the refrigerator every time she feels hungry. But these cautions are by no means limited to people with diabetes—such dietary excesses would be unhealthy for anyone. Unfortunately, large numbers of Americans have developed poor food habits, as evidenced by the fact that obesity is one of our leading health problems and that many of our most common diseases are associated with dietary excesses. But as the relationship between diet and total health becomes clearer, growing numbers of Americans are striving to improve their eating habits and to follow moderate, common-sense diets. While the diabetic patient must be more conscious of what he or she eats and its effect on blood glucose, the diet does not need to be greatly different from that consumed by any health-conscious person. Indeed, the overall dietary principles discussed in this chapter can be applied to the entire population.

To better understand the basics of meal planning, it's a good idea to start at the very beginning with a review of the basics of good nutrition. While some of this may seem elementary, Diabetes Self-Care dietitians have found that many patients and their families come to the program with numerous misconceptions and outdated concepts regarding diet and overall nutrition.

Foods fall into three general classifications of nutrients: carbohydrates, protein, and fats. A fourth element, fiber or roughage, is important in the human diet, but since it is not digested and metabolized it is not, strictly speaking, a nutrient. A good diet provides a balance of carbohydrates, protein, and fats, plus fiber, distributed in such a way that there are adequate vitamins and minerals to maintain good health and enough calories to provide energy and maintain proper weight. Most foods contain a combination of nutrients, with one predominating. For example, cereal grains contain all three, but complex carbohydrates (starch) predominate. Milk also contains all three, although the carbohydrates are in the form of a simple sugar, lactose. Most other animal products—meat, milk, eggs, poultry, or fish—contain protein and fat. All are needed in a healthy diet, but the typical American diet provides excessive fat, sugar, or simple carbohydrates, and calories.

Each class of nutrients has specific functions. Protein, for example, is used to build virtually every cell in the body and it is needed to make new tissue, repair the old, and maintain the body's chemical balance. It is essential to proper metabolism and almost all body functions. The protein that is not used for these functions is converted to glucose and used for energy or stored as body fat. Meat, fish, poultry, eggs, and other animal products are our major sources of protein, although protein also is found in grains, legumes, and seeds. Protein deficiency is rare in this country, although it may occur in people who follow a vegetarian diet that does not provide the proper balancing of grains, legumes, and seeds to form complete proteins.

Carbohydrates provide the body's major source of fuel or energy. There are two types of carbohydrates: the sugars, or simple carbohydrates, and starches, or complex carbohydrates. They are found in a variety of foods: fruits, vegetables, grains, legumes, and milk, which contains lactose, a sugar or simple carbohydrate. The body converts most carbohydrates to blood glucose, the body's major source of fuel or energy. The excess is stored as body fat.

Fats, the third essential nutrient, are perhaps the most misunderstood by the general public. The average person requires a relatively small amount of fat—about a tablespoon a day—but most Americans consume six to eight times that much. Most of this fat comes from animal sources: meat, whole milk, cheese, and egg yolks are common examples of high fat foods. These fats tend to be highly saturated, meaning they do not carry as much hydrogen as the other types of fatty acids, monounsaturated and polyunsaturated. Research has found that saturated fats tend to raise the level of blood cholesterol, a substance found in animal fats and that is also manufactured in the body. Although cholesterol is essential to many vital body functions, an excess in the blood is now considered to be a major factor in the development of atherosclerosis, the buildup of fatty deposits in the blood vessels, particularly the coronary arteries. Recent studies have found that lowering blood cholesterol can help prevent a heart attack —a factor that is particularly important to diabetic patients, who have a high incidence of coronary disease and heart attacks. Since the body manufactures all the cholesterol it needs, it is not necessary to consume it in the diet. In fact, we can get all the required fatty acids from monounsaturated or polyunsaturated fats, which tend to lower blood cholesterol. A certain amount of dietary fat has other benefits, however. It makes food taste better, and, since it is absorbed slowly from the digestive tract, it helps appease hunger. It is also important in the consumption and storage of fat-soluble vitamins. Some fat is used for body fuel, but most will be stored for future use.

Since diabetes is a disease that affects the body's ability to use and store blood glucose and since more than 90 percent of carbohydrates are converted to glucose, we tend to concentrate most on the effect of diabetes on carbohydrate metabolism. In reality, however, the disease also hinders the metabolism and storage of protein and fats. Normally, about half of the protein consumed is converted to glucose. In diabetes, however, the amount of protein (amino acids) metabolized by the muscles is reduced while the amount converted to glucose is increased. This altered protein metabolism explains, at least in part, the stunted growth of children with diabetes before the discovery of insulin. Although the effects of diabetes on fat metabolism are not as readily apparent as the effects on carbohydrates and protein, the disease also alters fat storage and use. For example, a lack of insulin increases the metabolism of stored body fat, which in turn leads to the buildup of ketone bodies, the highly acidic substances that are a by-product of fat metabolism. Diabetic people also have a high rate of cardiovascular disease, a fact attributed to the buildup of fatty deposits in the coronary arteries. People with diabetes tend to have high levels of triglycerides, one of the fatty substances that circulate in the blood, and many also have high blood cholesterol. Studies have found that insulin therapy and good control of blood glucose levels can normalize the elevated triglyceride and other blood lipids within a short time.

THE SELF-CARE APPROACH TO DIET

Over the centuries, a variety of dietary regimens have been recommended for people with diabetes. Ancient doctors knew that the urine of people with diabetes contained sugar, even though they did not fully understand that this was some of the glucose that the body was unable to metabolize. These early doctors also recognized that the intake of food had a profound effect on the disease. Thus, one of the earliest treatments was simply to withhold food to the point of starvation, which prompted one medical historian to observe that "many a diabetic stayed alive by stealing the bread denied him by his doctor." But through the years some doctors almost accidentally stumbled on dietary principles that are valid in the treatment of diabetes. Weight reduction and caloric restriction remain the major treatment of overweight type 2 diabetic patients who are producing insulin but either in inadequate amounts for their body weight or whose bodies are not fully using it.

Nearly two hundred years ago, a surgeon general in the British Royal Artillery, Dr. John Rollo, proposed a diet high in animal products for diabetics without realizing he was prescribing a high-protein, high-fat, low-carbohydrate diet. As you will soon see, a highly refined version of this diet is still recommended in the treatment of type 1 diabetes. Unfortunately, many other early dietary approaches were not as on-target as Dr. Rollo's and, very often, the regimens did more harm than good. Some early doctors, for example, thought their patients needed to replace the lost sugar and fed them large amounts of candy and other sweets, a tactic that compounded the problem.

Although diet is an important factor in controlling diabetes, people with the type 1 form of the disease also need insulin injections to metabolize their food. Indeed, the secret of diabetes control is mastering the technique of matching insulin and food, which is why diet is so important. Until recently, this was a relatively difficult task for many people with diabetes because they lacked the tools to tell them how well they were matching the two. The development of home self-monitoring of blood glucose now enables the diabetic patient to tell almost immediately whether the insulin and food intake are in balance and to take the proper corrective steps if they are not.

At the Diabetes Self-Care Program, patients are taught a total approach to diabetes control by learning the three major steps simultaneously—how to monitor their own blood glucose, how to plan a balanced diet that fits their food preferences and lifestyles, and how to match insulin with their individual meal plans. The dietary component starts with determining their total food needs in terms of calories and nutrients. To make it easier to calculate calories, serving portions, and nutrients, Self-Care dietitians use the metric system. This enables you to use nutritional labels on prepared foods and standard food charts, which are usually stated in grams. You begin by determining your approximate weight in kilograms, which can be done by dividing your weight in pounds by 2.2. For example, if you weigh 132 pounds, your weight in kilograms is about 60. This figure is important both in calculating your total food intake and your insulin dosage.

To determine about how many calories you should consume in an average day, you must consider several factors: What is your activity level? Are you about the right weight for your sex and frame (see the following table). What is your age? (Calorie requirements are highest for active, growing children and adolescents and lowest for older, relatively sedentary adults.) The following chart shows you the approximate number of calories per kilogram required by adults.

DESIRABLE WEIGHT FOR HEIGHT

Height (in shoes)	Small Frame	Medium Frame	Large Frame
MEN			
5'2"	112–120	118–129	126–141
5'3"	115–123	121–133	129–144
5'4"	118–126	124–136	132–148
5'5"	121–129	127–139	135–152
5'6"	124–133	130–143	138–156
5'7"	128–137	134–147	142–161
5'8"	132–141	138–152	147–166
5'9"	136–145	142–156	151–170
5'10"	140–150	146–160	155–174
5'11"	144–154	150–165	159–179
6'	148–158	154–170	164–184
6'1"	152–162	158–175	168–189
6'2"	156–167	162–180	173–194
6'3"	160–171	167–185	178–199
6'4"	164–175	172–190	182–204
WOMEN			
4'10"	92–98	96–101	104–119
4'11"	94–101	98–110	106–122
5'	96–104	101–113	109–125
5'1"	99–107	104–116	112–128
5'2"	102–110	107–119	115–131
5'3"	105–113	110–122	118–134

Height (in shoes)	Small Frame	Medium Frame	Large Frame
5'4"	108–116	113–126	121–138
5'5"	111–119	116–130	125–142
5'6"	114–123	120–135	129–146
5'7"	118–127	124–139	133–150
5'8"	122–131	128–143	137–154
5'9"	126–135	132–147	141–158
5'10"	130–140	136–151	145–163
5'11"	134–144	140–155	149–168
6'	138–148	144–159	153–173

Weight Status	Activity Level		
	Sedentary	Moderately Active	Very Active
Overweight	12–20	25	35
Normal	25	30	40
Underweight	30	35	45

If you are a sedentary office worker weighing 180 pounds (about 77 kilograms) and you should lose 15 pounds, you may be advised to calculate your caloric requirements at 20 calories per kilogram ($20 \times 77 = 1{,}540$ calories per day). If you are at your ideal body weight and are moderately active, you would strive for 30 calories per kilogram ($30 \times 77 = 2{,}310$). If you are at your normal weight and are training for a marathon, you would fall into the very active category and require 40 calories per kilogram ($40 \times 77 = 3{,}080$). (These figures are for adults; the following table gives the average daily caloric requirements for children.)

RECOMMENDED DAILY CALORIC INTAKE
FOR CHILDREN*

Age and Weight (Boys and Girls)	Calories
1 year (22 +/− 2 lbs)	1,000
2–3 years (30 +/− 5 lbs)	1,300
4–5 years (39 +/− 6 lbs)	1,700
6–9 years (56 +/− 15 lbs)	2,400
10–12 years (81 +/− 20 lbs)	2,700
13–15 years (108 +/− 27 lbs)	2,500–2,800

* Recommended Dietary Allowances, Revised 1980, National Research Council, National Academy of Sciences.

The next step is figuring how you should distribute your total calories among carbohydrates, protein, and fats. First, you should know that each gram of carbohydrates and protein equals 4 calories, while there are 9 calories in a gram of fat. The recommended distribution of nutrients for type 1 diabetics varies somewhat among the experts. For example, the American Diabetes Association recommends that 50 to 60 percent of the total calories come from carbohydrates, 15 to 20 percent come from protein, and 20 to 35 percent come from fats. The Cornell-Rockefeller physicians and dietitians who developed the Self-Care Program use a different distribution: 40 percent carbohydrates, 20 to 25 percent protein, and 35 to 40 percent fat. Dietitian Joan Choppin explains this difference: "In 1979, the American Diabetes and American Dietetic Associations recommended that dietary carbohydrate be increased over levels previously recommended, to 50 to 60 percent of total calories, with a corresponding reduction in fat and animal protein. This recommendation was based on increasing evidence from epidemiological studies linking coronary heart disease with diets high in total fat and/or saturated fats. The Cornell-Rockefeller approach advocates a somewhat lower carbohydrate allowance of 40 percent carbohydrate, 20 percent protein, and 40 percent fat. The lower carbohydrate level makes it easier to maintain blood glucose levels below 140 mg/dl, and the long-term advantage of tight blood glucose control appears to outweigh the risk that may result from a higher fat and/or protein content."

Still, program nutritionists caution patients to pay attention to the sources of fat and protein calories. For example, Barbara Turro teaches patients to concentrate on polyunsaturated fats and to emphasize complex carbohydrates that contain vegetable protein and fiber. And, in keeping with the total approach of the Self-Care Program, patients also are given an exercise program designed to promote cardiovascular health and fitness—an approach that many researchers feel helps keep both weight and blood cholesterol at healthier levels.

As in any eating plan for people with type 1 diabetes, Self-Care patients are taught to distribute the total number of calories throughout the day. The meals are timed to coincide with peak effectiveness of insulin. For most patients, this means eating three meals and several snacks at regular times during the day. More freedom can be gained, however, by experimenting with food, exercise, and insulin.

During the learning period, Self-Care patients plan for three meals and two or three snacks, timed to match three insulin injections. Once the diabetes is under good control and the patient feels confident in his or her ability to anticipate and solve problems, experimentation with different foods or routines is encouraged. "Most of us tend to be creatures of habit," Dr. Peterson notes, "eating our meals at fairly regular times and living according to a set schedule or pattern. But there are times when a person may want to alter the routine, or special circumstances like a traffic jam or sudden trip may intervene to change the daily pattern. We want our patients to feel confident that they can handle these circumstances."

To match food and insulin, you have to know when the insulin will be at its most effective levels and when the food you eat is likely to be converted to blood glucose. While a number of factors can affect both, there are specific guidelines to follow. Important points to remember are:

- What kind of insulin are you taking, how long does it take to start acting, when does it peak, and how long is it effective? (These questions are discussed in detail in Chapter 5.)
- How many calories should you consume in a day and what percentage of them should be from carbohydrates?

With this information, you can develop a working meal plan. As a first step, calculate insulin dosages as described in Chapter 5. The next step involves calculating how much food you should eat during the course of a day, and how you should distribute it. To find total calorie requirements, refer to the chart on page 53. If your weight is normal and you are moderately active, you can have 30 calories per kilogram. To see how this works, let's do the calculations for a moderately active male patient weighing 158 pounds, or 72 kilograms. The total caloric allowance would be 2,160 per day. He is going to consume 40 percent of these calories (864) in carbohydrates; 25 percent (540) in protein, and 35 percent (756) in fats. To make calculations easier, we figure out how many grams of each nutrient he should eat. Since there are 4 calories in a gram of carbohydrates or protein and 9 calories in a gram of fat, this means that our patient should eat 216 grams of carbohydrates, 135 grams of protein, and 84 grams of fat. (It is not necessary to be too rigid about these amounts; the idea is to learn the boundaries in which you can keep your blood sugar in the normal range.)

Ordinarily, a Self-Care patient on three injections of a combination of an intermediate-acting (e.g., NPH) and fast-acting (e.g., Regular) insulin would distribute these 216 grams of carbohydrates over three meals and three snacks, or along the following lines:

Breakfast	10% or 22 grams of carbohydrates
Midmorning snack	5% or 11 grams
Lunch	30% or 65 grams
Midafternoon snack	10% or 22 grams

Dinner   30% or 65 grams
Evening snack   5% or 11 grams
Before-bed snack   10% or 22 grams

Let's suppose that this patient exercises for about a half hour every afternoon. He might find he needs a somewhat larger afternoon snack, and that only one after-dinner, before-bed snack seems to carry him through the night without his blood sugar going too low during the night. This is revealed by his diary of blood sugar measurements, insulin injections, and food intake. (See Chapter 4 for details on how to keep your own Self-Care Program diary.)

A patient who is maintained on a slow-acting (e.g., Ultralente) and Regular insulin would follow a somewhat different meal and snack plan, with 10 percent of the total carbohydrates consumed at breakfast, 40 percent at lunch, 40 percent at dinner, and 10 percent in a before-bed snack.

To match insulin and food, you must know how long it takes the foods you eat to appear as blood glucose in your body. Simple carbohydrates are converted to blood glucose the fastest: 90 to 100 percent of carbohydrates is converted to glucose. Simple carbohydrates, such as lactose (milk sugar), sucrose (table sugar), or glucose, begin to have an almost immediate effect on blood glucose which will peak in fifteen to thirty minutes after you eat these foods. Complex carbohydrates or starches take longer, with blood glucose peaking sixty to ninety minutes after consumption. Fiber slows the process, which is one reason why high-fiber foods should be included in your meals and snacks.

About 50 to 60 percent of protein is converted to blood glucose, but the process takes longer than the metabolism of carbohydrates. Glucose from protein begins to rise sixty to ninety minutes after eating and peaks in about three hours. Very little fat, less than 10 percent, is converted to glucose, so it has little or no effect on blood sugar.

In the beginning, Self-Care Program patients carefully measure and weigh all their food. Close attention is paid to nutritional labels, which specify grams of carbohydrates, protein, and fat. If nutritional labels are not available, you can consult a number of books: *Food Values of Portions Commonly Used* by Jean A. T. Pennington and Helen Nichols Church (Harper Colophon Books) is one used by Self-Care dietitians. This may sound tedious, but in a few days you will find that you can tell by looking at a serving about how many grams of a particular nutrient it contains. For most people, a few grams either way does not make much difference, but for the person with type 1 diabetes, miscalculating by as little as 20 grams of simple carbohydrates—the amount in a medium-sized orange, 3 ounces of seedless grapes, or 1 ounce of raisins, for example—can have a considerable effect on blood glucose if there is not enough insulin present to handle it. This is why it is important to know about how much insulin will be required to cover a particular food or meal. In general, you should take 1 unit of insulin for every 10 grams of carbohydrates, although a number of factors may alter this.

A Word About Breakfast

Starting the day with blood glucose under control is an important tenet of the Diabetes Self-Care Program, and for many diabetic patients, this may mean sharply reducing or even delaying breakfast. A hearty breakfast is, in the eyes of many Americans, in the same class as motherhood and apple pie. Most nutrition books urge people to "start the day right" by consuming about a third of the day's total calories for breakfast. In the past, many diabetes dietary plans offered similar advice, advocating relatively big breakfasts that included relatively large amounts of carbohydrates. For example, the following menu is one that has been recommended for diabetic patients:

Food	Grams of carbohydrates
4 ounces orange juice	14
3/4 cup cornflakes or other unsweetened cereal	16

1/2 banana	11
8 ounces skim milk	12
2 slices whole wheat toast	24
Total carbohydrates	77

As Dr. Jovanovic points out, this breakfast contains about a third of the total daily allotment of carbohydrates recommended by the Diabetes Self-Care Program for a 72-kilogram adult, and more than three times the 22 grams slated for breakfast. "I could almost guarantee that this breakfast will send blood sugar soaring, and will put the patient with diabetes out of control for the entire day," she says.

There is a clear rationale for a breakfast that is relatively low in carbohydrates. At about 3 A.M., the blood glucose level of most diabetic patients is at its lowest point of the twenty-four hours. Then, as the counterregulatory "wake-up" hormones come into play, the body becomes more insulin-resistant and blood sugar begins to drift up; it may be 100 mg/dl or higher by the time you wake up. If you get up at about 7 A.M. with a blood glucose over 100 mg/dl, take an injection of Regular and NPH insulin, and eat the above breakfast at 7:30, the blood sugar may be 300 mg/dl or higher before the prebreakfast insulin peaks. "Obviously, this is a situation you want to avoid," Dr. Jovanovic comments. The easiest strategy is to eat a low-carbohydrate breakfast.

If you need a fair amount of food to get started in the morning, plan a breakfast that is high in protein, which takes about three hours to be converted to blood glucose. An egg or cottage cheese are possible high-protein choices. Avoid fruit and other sources of simple sugar for breakfast; instead, eat complex carbohydrates that also contain fiber (for example, oatmeal flavored with spices or an artificial sweetener). Other strategies might include getting up earlier, injecting your insulin, and then waiting an hour or so to eat. If the waking blood sugar is high, a few minutes of exercise after taking your insulin and before eating breakfast also will help keep it in check.

Morning fasting blood sugar that is consistently too high or too low also may be a sign to adjust the insulin dosage. Breakfast is covered by the peaking of the before-bed NPH and the onset of action from the Regular insulin. But a fasting blood glucose of 120 to 140 mg/dl is a sign to add extra Regular insulin to your prebreakfast injection. In general, Self-Care physicians recommend the following insulin adjustments based on the before-breakfast blood glucose levels. Start by adjusting the morning Regular dosage. If the fasting blood glucose levels are too high or too low for two days in a row, adjust the before-bed basal insulin dosage as well as the morning injection.

Blood Glucose	Insulin Adjustments	
(mg/dl)	*Morning Regular*	*Before-Bed NPH*
Less than 70	Decrease 2 units	Decrease 2 units
70–100	Leave as is	Leave as is
100–140	Increase 2 units	Increase 2 units
Over 140	Increase 4 units	Increase 4 units
		and consult doctor

Similarly, if the before-dinner blood sugar is below 70 mg/dl, it may be an indication to lower the before-breakfast NPH and adjust the before-dinner Regular. However, you should get your fasting glucose under control before attempting to adjust other insulin dosages. Most people find that once their mornings are normal, the rest of the day will be easier to control.

USING FOOD IN PROBLEM SOLVING

From time to time, most people with diabetes will experience an episode of low blood sugar, or hypoglycemia. The cause may be too much insulin, too little food, a response to exercise, a delayed meal, or other circumstance. The blood sugar can be brought back up by eating, but care must be taken to prevent a bounce, in which the blood sugar rises quickly and then falls again. Instead, the goal should be to raise the blood sugar to the desired level and then maintain it there.

· The type and amount of food consumed will determine whether you achieve this goal; the secret is knowing how much a particular food will raise the blood sugar. The strategy recommended for Self-Care patients is to combine a simple sugar with protein and/or complex carbohydrates. This will provide the needed fast rise and will also give the slower, steady maintenance as the protein or complex carbohydrate is converted. As noted earlier, milk is an ideal food to counter hypoglycemia because it contains lactose, a simple sugar, and protein. An 8-ounce glass of milk should increase blood sugar 25 to 30 mg/dl in about fifteen minutes.

If the blood sugar is very low, say 40 mg/dl, more simple carbohydrates may be needed. Dr. Jovanovic suggests drinking 4 ounces of orange juice, followed a few minutes later by a glass of milk or a slice of bread with cheese. An 8-ounce glass of orange juice may raise blood glucose about 100 mg/dl; this may be too rapid an increase and may produce a bounce. If milk is not available and you eat other sources of sugar to counter the hypoglycemia—for example, candy, raisins, an apple, etc.—try to add a protein food to achieve the same effect you would get with milk.

Of course, low blood sugar is not the only problem commonly encountered by diabetic patients: high blood glucose or hyperglycemia is an even more common problem, especially in people whose disease is out of control. As repeatedly emphasized in this book, the goal of all patients with diabetes is to normalize blood glucose levels into the gray zone, which is between 50 and 150 mg/dl. Most people can achieve this with careful self-monitoring, multiple insulin injections, and proper timing of eating and exercise. Self-Care patients measure their blood sugar before eating; if the levels are on the high side, the patients are instructed to wait until the glucose is below 120 mg/dl. "If you don't want to delay eating for too long, you can bring the blood sugar down by a few minutes of exercise," Dr. Jovanovic points out.

Many diabetic patients, especially those whose disease is not well controlled, feel hungry a good deal of the time. Lowering blood sugar will diminish these feelings of hunger. In addition, you can concentrate on foods that will promote a feeling of fullness without greatly raising blood glucose. A salad of fresh vegetables with an oil and vinegar dressing will provide some simple carbohydrates, but the fiber will slow the conversion to glucose. As noted earlier, foods high in fat will satisfy hunger longer than carbohydrates because of their slow absorption time. High-fat foods do have certain disadvantages: they are high in calories and animal or other saturated fats that may increase cholesterol levels. But there are now many food products that use polyunsaturated fats or foods that add bulk and a mixture of fat, protein, and complex carbohydrates. A chicken or tuna salad sandwich or pasta dishes such as lasagna are examples of foods that provide a balance of nutrients.

SAMPLE MENUS

The following menus are built around carbohydrate allowances and illustrate the wide variety of common foods that can be worked into a diabetic's diet. Self-Care dietitians repeatedly stress that, for the most part, people with type 1 diabetes can enjoy the same foods served to other members of the household. But it would be folly to think you can approach food with the same sense of abandon as the nondiabetic. Problem-free eating requires proper timing, planning, and insulin coverage. You will soon learn how various foods and circumstances affect blood glucose. By following the Self-Care (or your doctor's) guidelines for matching food and insulin and adjusting insulin dosages, you can acquire a high degree of eating flexibility.

EATING OUT

Many people with diabetes, including those who have mastered matching insulin and food at home, find they are stymied when it comes to eating out, especially if it is an out of the ordinary occasion. If a daily routine includes eating lunch or some other meal at work, this becomes a part of the normal regimen. But a special occasion such as a dinner party or a festive evening at a restaurant is not a day-to-day activity and may require extra planning. All too often, the diabetic patient in such a situation misjudges and winds up out of control for several days. This does not mean you should avoid the pleasure of eating out; if you know how to plan for such events, they can be managed without incident

Just knowing when and how to take your insulin can help prevent many problems. Dr. Jovanovic sometimes cites an incident from her own experience that illustrates the kind of problems a person with diabetes should know how to anticipate. She had been invited to a dinner party and she mistakenly assumed that dinner would be served near the appointed hour. When it seemed that dinner was in the offing, she took a larger than usual injection of insulin in anticipation of eating a big meal complete with a rich dessert. But, as often happens, dinner was late and the snack tray of fresh vegetables, cheese dips, and other tasty tidbits did not offer the high amount of carbohydrates she had anticipated. "I knew that I was beginning to experience an insulin reaction, so I finally asked my hostess for a glass of milk and some orange juice," she recalls. "And from that experience, I learned never to take my insulin until the food is being served."

According to Dr. Jovanovic, there are two reasons for waiting until your meal is being served. "First, you know for sure that the food will be available when you need it," she explains. "And you will be able to judge the actual size of the portions and take the right amount of insulin." To avoid having too fast a rise in blood glucose before your insulin starts to act, you can dawdle a bit over your salad or some other complex carbohydrate first, and then eat your protein course. The fiber in the salad will slow the rise in blood sugar, and the complex carbohydrates take longer than simple sugar to be converted to glucose.

Many people feel uncomfortable taking an insulin injection in a public place. As one Self-Care patient explained: "I usually go to the restroom, but even this is not always satisfactory. If someone sees you with a syringe, they invariably associate it with an illegal drug." To avoid such situations, Dr. Jovanovic teaches patients how to discretely inject themselves at the table. She concedes that this is not the way patients are taught to make injections, and "I wouldn't want my patients to do it all the time." The important thing is to be prepared with adequate insulin and to time its administration with your meal. A bit of rule bending regarding the method of injection is acceptable if it makes you more comfortable and if it does not hinder the insulin action.

Patients who use an insulin pump have a special advantage because it is relatively easy to administer the proper amount of insulin to cover the food. Regardless of the method of administration, you should plan to measure your blood glucose about three hours after a meal. If it is high, you can take a bit of extra insulin to bring it to the desired level. (See Chapter 5 for more details on how to do this.)

Of course, one of the pitfalls experienced by anyone, including nondiabetics, who frequents fine restaurants with a wide array of foods is the temptation to overeat. Most restaurants serve overly generous portions and often the food is prepared with high-calorie sauces and extras. If you eat out often, you should learn to judge portion size and to develop tactics that will help you eat in moderation and still enjoy the experience. Fortunately, a growing number of restaurants, including such fashionable ones as New York's Four Seasons, are making extra efforts to accommodate their health- and weight-conscious patrons by offering delicious yet light foods. Also, restaurants that prepare each dish to order (as opposed to fast-food restaurants where food usually is mass-produced) usually will cook food according to individual requests. Some may require advance notice, for example, to prepare a special dessert with a sugar substitute. Many people hesitate to ask a chef to depart from the usual way of preparing food and they often are surprised to learn that most will acceed to their diners' wishes. Remember, you are paying for what you eat and you have the right to have it cooked according to the way you want.

THE QUESTION OF ALCOHOL

Many misconceptions persist about alcohol consumption. Many people with diabetes avoid alcohol completely, often in the mistaken belief that even a small amount of wine or other alcoholic beverage will disrupt glucose control. Others confess to an occasional drink, but feel guilty about it. While excessive consumption of alcohol is not good for anyone, there is no reason why a diabetic whose disease is under good control cannot now and then enjoy an occasional meal-time drink. Contrary to popular belief, there is no evidence that a mealtime glass of wine or other alcoholic beverage can raise havoc with glucose levels, but like so many facets of a diabetic patient's life, a good deal depends on knowing how and when to drink.

Self-Care dietitians caution their patients to time having a drink to coincide with a meal or a snack. The effect on blood sugar depends on the composition of the drink: the calories in distilled spirits, such as whiskey, gin, or vodka, come mostly from ethanol, which does not require insulin for metabolism. But wine, beer, and certain mixed drinks also contain carbohydrates that are metabolized the same as any simple sugar. Port, sweet wines, and liqueurs should be avoided by diabetic patients because of their very high sugar content. Also, the best choices for mixers are those that are low in sugar; diet soft drinks, club soda, seltzer, or water, which would include sparkling or mineral waters. Light beers and wines have fewer calories from both alcohol and carbohydrates than regular types; dry wines also have little or no sugar. In any event, an alcoholic beverage should not contribute more than 6 percent of the day's total calories. The following table summarizes the alcohol, carbohydrate, and caloric content of common alcoholic beverages.

GUIDE TO ALCOHOLIC BEVERAGES

Beverage	Measure (ounces)	Alcohol (grams)	Carbohydrates (grams)	Calories
Ale	12	13.1	12.0	147
Beer	12	13.3	15.8	150
Beer, light	12	12.1	2.8	100
WINES				
Champagne	4	11.0	3.0	84
Red	4	10.0	0.5	85
Muscatel/port	3½	15.0	14.0	158
Dry white	4	10.5	4.0	85
Dessert	4	15.3	7.7	137
COCKTAILS				
Eggnog	4	15.0	18.0	335
Gin, rum, vodka, scotch	4	12–16	0	277
Martini	3½	18.5	0.3	140
Manhattan	3½	19.2	7.9	164
CORDIALS				
Benedictine	2/3	6.6	6.6	75
Brandy	1	10.5	7.0	85

Sources: Janet McDonald, "Whiskey or Water," *Diabetes Forecast,* November–December 1980, pp. 42–43, and Jean A. T. Pennington and Helen Nichols Church, *Food Values of Portions Commonly Used,* 13th ed. New York: Harper/Colophon Books, 1980.

SUMMING UP

To normalize blood sugar, the diabetic patient must follow a three-pronged approach: diet, insulin, and exercise. All are interrelated; learning to match insulin with food and exercise is the key to success. The dietary approach followed by the Diabetes Self-Care Program is somewhat different from the exchange system with which many diabetic patients are familiar. But once you master the concept of building meals and snacks around a carbohydrate allowance and dividing total calories among both meals and nutrient groups, it becomes a relatively simple task. The Self-Care approach also offers greater flexibility and lets you experiment with foods and lifestyle accommodations.

SAMPLE MENUS

Self-Care patients are given choices similar to those they may find in any cafeteria; the menus and recipes also can be adapted for home use. Patients eat breakfast before coming to the center, making their food selections according to personal preference and their calorie and carbohydrate allowances. In selecting foods from a menu, patients are instructed to measure serving sizes using a scale or measuring cups until they can accurately estimate a serving. The grams of carbohydrates, protein, and fat and total calories are calculated in the accompanying recipes; in real practice, patients would consult a guide such as *Food Values of Portions Commonly Used.*

Patients are by no means limited to these food choices; the menus are designed to indicate the variety of foods available. Self-Care Program dietitians often make last-minute changes in menus to accommodate the food preferences of patients. "We emphasize that people with diabetes can eat almost anything they like so long as they know how to plan for it and adjust their insulin and exercise accordingly," explains Barbara Turro, one of the program dietitians. There are a number of good cookbooks specifically for people with diabetes, but, as Turro states, "Most favorite family recipes can be adapted by using sugar substitutes where appropriate and balancing the menu to provide the proper percentages of carbohydrates, protein, and fats."

MENUS

Monday

LUNCH
Spaghetti with meatballs
Tossed salad
Apple
Beverage

DINNER
Chicken paprikash*
Broccoli
Brown rice
Tossed salad
Cheese
Beverage

Tuesday

LUNCH
Onion soup
Salmon salad
  or omelette
Tossed salad
Beverage

DINNER
Rolled flounder
Baked potato
Zucchini
Tossed salad
Stewed pear*
Beverage

Wednesday

LUNCH
Lentil soup
Tossed salad
Cheese
Beverage

DINNER
Meat loaf*
Baked potato
Steamed cabbage/peppers
Tossed salad
Strawberry fluff*
Beverage

* Recipes included.

Thursday

LUNCH
Anne's soufflé
macaroni and cheese*
Tossed salad
Fresh fruit
Beverage

DINNER
Cornish hen*
Brown rice
Asparagus
Tossed salad
Pineapple gelatin*
Beverage

Friday

LUNCH
Corn chowder
Sliced turkey
Tossed salad
Fruit cup
Beverage

DINNER
Beef stew*
Anne's easy biscuits*
Spinach salad
Melon
Beverage

Weekend Menus

Although the Diabetes Self-Care Program serves meals only on weekdays, dietitians are available to help patients plan special menus for weekends, entertaining, and other occasions. Following are some sample menus developed with Barbara Turro.

SATURDAY SUPPER
Anne's meat lasagna*
Green beans with almonds
Orange slices
Beverage

SUNDAY DINNER
Onion soup
Veal piccata*
Dilled carrots

Tossed salad
Rice pudding*
Beverage

PARTY DINNER
Gazpacho*
Lamb curry*
Couscous
Broccoli
Chocolate chiffon mold*
Beverage

RECIPES

GAZPACHO*

1 clove garlic, peeled
1 pound ripe tomatoes
1 1/2 pounds (about 2 large)
    cucumbers
1 cup finely diced green
    pepper
3/4 cup finely diced celery
1/2 cup finely diced onion
2 cups tomato juice or
    cocktail vegetable juice
1 tablespoon vegetable oil

1 cup cold water
3 dashes Tabasco sauce
1 teaspoon salt
1/2 teaspoon coarsely ground
    black pepper
1/2 cup seasoned croutons, for
    garnish
Chopped fresh parsley, for
    garnish

Crush garlic in the bottom of a 2 1/2-quart bowl. Core tomatoes and discard cores and seeds; finely dice tomatoes. Pare cucumbers, cut lengthwise in eighths, discard centers and seeds; finely dice remaining cucumber. Measure all ingredients except croutons and parsley into the large bowl on top of the garlic. Mix thoroughly. Cover bowl tightly and chill for 2 hours or longer. Serve soup in chilled bowls garnished with croutons and parsley. 9 servings of about 10 ounces each.

Nutritive values per serving: Carbohydrates 10 grams
                               Protein   2 grams
                               Fat   2 grams
                               Calories   66

VEAL PICCATA*

2 tablespoons flour
1/2 teaspoon salt
1/4 teaspoon pepper
11/4 pound veal scallops, very
  thinly sliced
3 tablespoons margarine

1 lemon with rind, very thinly
  sliced crosswise
1/3 cup dry white wine
1/3 cup lemon juice
2 tablespoons chopped fresh
  parsley, for garnish

Combine the flour, salt, and pepper; sprinkle on both sides of the veal scallops. Heat 1½ tablespoons margarine over medium heat in a very large frying pan and quickly sauté half of the veal 2 to 3 minutes until the edges brown slightly; repeat process with remaining 1½ tablespoons margarine and veal. Remove meat from pan and set it aside. To the pan drippings add three quarters of the lemon slices, the wine, and lemon juice; scrape drippings into this liquid, mix well, and bring mixture to a boil. Return veal to pan and cook gently 2 to 3 minutes to blend flavors. Serve immediately on warm platter. Garnish with remaining lemon slices and chopped parsley. 4 servings.

Nutritive values per serving: Carbohydrates 9 grams
                               Protein   28 grams
                               Fat   20 grams
                               Calories   328

BEEF STEW*

1/4 cup flour
1 1/4 teaspoon salt
1/8 teaspoon black pepper
1/4 teaspoon dry mustard
1 1/4 pounds top round steak,
　　1 inch thick
1 tablespoon vegetable oil
2 1/2 cups water
1 teaspoon Worcestershire
　　sauce

2 cups pared, quartered, and
　　sliced potatoes (about 13
　　ounces)
1 cup sliced onions
1 cup carrots, sliced crosswise
1/2 teaspoon dillweed
　　(optional)

Preheat oven to 350° F (180° C). Combine flour, salt, pepper, and mustard in a paper bag. Trim off all fat around outside of round steak; cut meat into 1-inch cubes. Shake meat cubes in the paper bag with flour, a few at a time, until they are well coated. Heat oil in a large frying pan; brown meat cubes over medium heat, turning with tongs until meat is evenly browned. Transfer meat cubes to a 2 1/2-quart casserole; set aside. Sprinkle seasoned flour remaining in paper bag into the fat remaining in the frying pan; stir vigorously until smooth and mixed. Add water very slowly and stir; add Worcestershire sauce. Cook and stir until smooth; pour on top of meat in casserole. Cover and cook in oven for 2 hours. Mix vegetables and dillweed into meat, cover, and cook in oven for 1 more hour, or until meat and vegetables are tender. 4 (1-cup) servings.

Nutritive values per serving:	Carbohydrates	25 grams
	Protein	26 grams
	Fat	18 grams
	Calories	366
	Sodium	816 milligrams

CHICKEN PAPRIKASH

*1 chicken (2½ pounds), cut
in quarters
2 tablespoons olive oil
1 clove garlic, crushed
1 cup chopped onions
1½ tablespoons paprika
(more or less, as desired)*

*½ teaspoon ground cumin
2 cups chicken broth
½ teaspoon salt
1 cup cross-sliced carrots
2 tablespoons tomato paste*

Wipe chicken pieces with a damp paper towel and set aside. Heat oil in a deep 10- or 12-inch frying pan. Add garlic and onion and cook gently over low heat, stirring occasionally, until they are a very light golden color. Add paprika and cumin and continue cooking about 1 minute. Place chicken pieces in pan with skin side down. Add chicken broth, salt, and carrots; cover pan tightly and simmer over low heat for 25 minutes. Stir in the tomato paste. Turn chicken pieces, cover again, and simmer over low heat for 25 to 30 minutes, or until chicken is tender. 4 servings.

Nutritive values per serving:

Carbohydrates	10 grams	
Protein	34 grams	
Fat	17 grams	
Calories	329	

MEAT LOAF*

*1 beef bouillon cube
½ cup boiling water
2 slices bread, finely
crumbled
1½ pounds 85% lean
ground beef
2 medium eggs, slightly
beaten*

*½ cup finely chopped onion
¼ cup finely chopped celery
2 teaspoons Worcestershire
sauce
1 tablespoon catsup*

Preheat oven to 350° F (180° C). Line a shallow 8-inch-square baking pan with foil. Dissolve beef bouillon cube in boiling water in a large bowl. Add all other ingredients except the catsup and blend well with a fork. Turn onto foil in pan and, with your hands, shape quickly into a 6 × 4½ × 2-inch loaf. With the dull edge of a knife make a crisscross pattern across the top; spread catsup on top. Cover loaf with a tent of foil that does not touch the top. Bake for 45 minutes. Remove foil; bake uncovered for another 45 minutes. Remove from oven and cool in pan for 2 to 3 minutes before serving. Using this molded method instead of a loaf pan allows the fat to drain from the loaf, whereas a loaf pan retains fat.

Nutritive values per serving:

1 large slice	Carbohydrates	7 grams	
(4½ × 2 × 1 inch)	Protein	26 grams	
	Fat	16 grams	
	Calories	276	
1 medium slice	Carbohydrates	5 grams	
(4½ × 2 × ¾ inch)	Protein	20 grams	
	Fat	12 grams	
	Calories	208	

ANNE'S SOUFFLÉ MACARONI AND CHEESE

1½ cup skim milk
6 ounces skim milk
American cheese
4 ounces grated Parmesan
cheese

2 eggs, lightly beaten
1 cup macaroni, uncooked
4 tablespoons margarine

Preheat oven to 350° F (180° C). Heat milk to just below scalding. Add cheeses and slowly add eggs, a little at a time, stirring constantly to prevent coagulating. Stir over low heat until cheeses are melted. Cook macaroni according to package instructions; drain, stir in margarine. Put in baking dish; pour cheese sauce over top and bake for 15 minutes. 10 (½ cup) servings.

Nutritive values per serving:

Carbohydrates	9	grams
Protein	11	grams
Fat	10	grams
Calories	170	

ANNE'S MEAT LASAGNA

8 ounces lean ground beef
1 large onion, diced
2 cloves garlic
1 (16-ounce) can whole tomatoes
1 (6-ounce) can tomato paste
1 teaspoon dried basil
½ teaspoon dried oregano

1 teaspoon salt
½ teaspoon parsley flakes
8 ounces lasagna noodles, uncooked
8 ounces mozzarella cheese, part skim milk
2 ounces grated Parmesan cheese

Brown beef with onion and garlic, drain off excess fat. Add tomatoes and tomato paste, basil, oregano, salt, and parsley flakes; simmer, uncovered, for 30 minutes, stirring occasionally.

Preheat oven to 350° F (180° C). Cook lasagna noodles according to package instructions. In a 12-inch square baking pan, alternate layers of meat sauce, noodles, and cheese. Bake, uncovered, for 30 minutes. 12 servings.

Nutritive values per serving:

Carbohydrates	20	grams
Protein	15	grams
Fat	9	grams
Calories	221	

ROCK CORNISH HENS*

1 1/2 tablespoon margarine   1/2 cup dry white wine
1 teaspoon salt   1/4 cup grape juice,
1/4 teaspoon pepper   unsweetened
2 Rock Cornish hens, about   1/2 cup seedless green or red
    1 1/4 pounds each   grapes, cut in half
1/2 cup chicken broth

Melt margarine in a saucepan; add salt and pepper. Split hens and place in shallow baking pan, skin side up. Baste with margarine mixture. Roast hens, uncovered, for 1 1/4 hours, or until tender and brown. When hens are done, remove them from pan. Pour drippings into a small saucepan, add chicken broth, wine, and grape juice. Simmer 15 minutes, or until volume is reduced to 3/4 cup. Add grapes and cook 2 minutes over moderate heat. Put hens on heated serving dish and pour grape mixture over them. 4 servings.

Nutritive values per serving: Carbohydrates   8 grams
                               Protein   25 grams
                               Fat   8 grams
                               Calories   204

LAMB CURRY*

2 tablespoons margarine   1 tablespoon curry powder or
2 cups coarsely chopped   to taste
    onions   1/4 teaspoon ground ginger
1 large clove garlic, minced   1 teaspoon salt
1 1/2 pounds boneless lean   1 1/2 cups hot chicken broth
    lamb, cut into 1-inch   1 (16-ounce) can tomatoes
    cubes   1 cup (100 grams) cubed,
3 tablespoons flour   pared apples

Melt margarine in a large, deep frying pan. Add onions, garlic, and lamb and cook over medium heat, stirring frequently, until meat is browned all over. Remove lamb and onions with a slotted spoon and set aside. Combine flour, curry powder, ginger, and salt and stir into remaining fat in frying pan; blend well. Add hot chicken broth slowly, stirring constantly, until smooth and beginning to bubble. Cut tomatoes into bite-sized pieces; add tomatoes and tomato liquid, lamb, onions, and apples to mixture in pan. Stir to blend; bring to a simmer. Cover and cook over low heat about 45 minutes, or until meat is tender, stirring occasionally. Serve with rice. 6 servings.

Nutritive values per serving:

Carbohydrates	15	grams
Protein	25	grams
Fat	10	grams
Sodium	742	milligrams
Calories	250	

ANNE'S EASY BISCUITS

1/2 cup shortening   *2 cups self-rising flour*
2/3 cup 2% milk   *2 egg yolks*

Preheat oven to 350° F (180° C). Soften shortening. Add milk, flour, and egg yolks. Blend lightly. Roll out on floured board to 1/2-inch thickness. Use small glass or cookie cutter to make 15 (2-inch) biscuits. Place about 2 inches apart on lightly greased cookie sheet for about 10 minutes, or until golden brown.

Nutritional values per biscuit:

Carbohydrates	12	grams
Protein	2	grams
Fat	7	grams
Calories	112	

POACHED PEARS*

5 small, just underripe pears
(d'Anjou, Bartlett, or Bosc)
—1 pound total
3 1/2 cups water
2 tablespoons lemon juice
2 teaspoons imitation rum
flavor

1 teaspoon pure vanilla
extract
1 1/4 teaspoon pure orange
flavor
Artificial sweetener to
substitute for 2 1/2
tablespoons sugar

Pare, halve lengthwise, and core the pears; the total weight of the 10 halves will be approximately 330 grams (11 ounces). Put prepared pear halves, water, and lemon juice in a saucepan. Bring to a boil, turn heat down, and let simmer gently 20 to 22 minutes, or until pears are tender but firm. Remove from heat. Lift pears out carefully with a spoon and place in a pint jar or bowl. Add all flavorings and artificial sweetener to hot liquid; stir to blend well. Pour on top of pears. Cover tightly. Cool at room temperature, then chill for several hours or overnight in refrigerator. 5 servings.

Nutritive values per serving: Carbohydrates   10 grams
                                Calories   40

PINEAPPLE GELATIN*

2 teaspoons unflavored
gelatin
1/4 cup cold water
1/2 cup boiling water
1 teaspoon lemon juice
1 1/4 cups unsweetened
pineapple juice

Artificial sweetener to
substitute for 3 teaspoons
sugar
Strawberries, for garnish
(optional)

Soak gelatin in cold water. Add boiling water and lemon juice and stir to dissolve. Add pineapple juice and artificial sweetener; stir to dissolve. Chill until partially set, stirring occasionally. Spoon into a

2-cup serving dessert bowl or 4 individual dessert dishes. Chill until set. A pretty garnish of a whole or sliced strawberry on each may be added. 4 servings.

Nutritive values per serving:
Carbohydrates	11	grams
Protein	1	gram
Sodium	1	milligram
Calories	48	

STRAWBERRY FLUFF*

1/4 cup cold water
1 tablespoon unflavored
gelatin
1 tablespoon lemon juice
Artificial sweetener to
substitute for 10 teaspoons
sugar

1/4 teaspoon pure orange
flavor
1 pint (2 cups) fresh
strawberries
3 egg whites, at room
temperature
1/8 teaspoon salt

Measure water, gelatin, lemon juice, artificial sweetener, and orange flavor into a blender. Wash strawberries and remove hulls; set aside 1/2 cup berries. Cut remaining 11/2 cups berries in quarters and add to mixture in blender. Cover; turn blender to high speed for about 30 seconds, or until mixture is well blended. In a bowl, beat egg whites and salt until stiff but not dry. Fold strawberry mixture carefully into egg whites; blend well. Slice remaining berries. Put a few slices in the bottom of each of 6 individual serving dishes, then a layer of strawberry mixture, then more strawberry slices, more mixture, and finish with a few strawberry slices on top as garnish. Chill in refrigerator until firm. 6 (2/3-cup) servings.

Nutritive values per serving:
Carbohydrates	5	grams
Protein	3	grams
Sodium	66	milligrams
Calories	32	

RICE PUDDING*

2 cups skim milk
2 medium eggs, beaten
2 tablespoons sugar (or
    equivalent amount of
    artificial sweetener if
    desired)
1/4 teaspoon salt

1/4 teaspoon cinnamon
1 teaspoon pure vanilla
    extract
1 cup (145 grams) cold
    cooked rice
2 tablespoons seedless raisins

Preheat oven to 350° F (180° C). Coat a 1-quart casserole with shortening or vegetable cooking spray. Scald (heat) milk in the top of a double boiler over simmering water. Combine eggs, sugar, salt, cinnamon, and vanilla. Pour hot milk on top slowly, stirring to mix well. Spread rice in the bottom of the casserole; scatter raisins evenly over rice; pour milk mixture carefully on top. Place casserole in pan of hot water with hot water coming almost up to the top of the casserole. Bake about 45 minutes, or until knife tip inserted in center comes out clean. Remove casserole from water and chill in refrigerator. This pudding may be served warm or chilled, as you prefer. 4 (3/4-cup) servings.

Nutritive values per serving:

Carbohydrates	24	grams
Protein	8	grams
Fat	3	grams
Sodium	355	milligrams
Calories	155	

CHOCOLATE CHIFFON MOLD*

*1 tablespoon unflavored
  gelatin
1/2 cup cold water
3 medium eggs, separated, at
  room temperature
1/4 cup (25 grams) dry
  unsweetened cocoa
1/8 teaspoon salt
1 cup skim milk*

*1 1/2 teaspoons pure vanilla
  extract
1/2 teaspoon pure chocolate
  extract
Artificial sweetener to
  substitute for 2/3 cup sugar
6 small ladyfingers (42
  grams)
1/8 teaspoon cream of tartar*

Soak gelatin in cold water. Beat egg yolks until light; add cocoa, salt, and milk; beat until smooth. Turn into the top of a double boiler. Cook over simmering water, stirring constantly until thick and smooth. Remove from heat. Add vanilla, chocolate extract, and artificial sweetener; mix well. Add chocolate mixture to gelatin and stir until gelatin is completely dissolved. Chill in refrigerator, stirring occasionally, until mixture sets to the consistency of unbeaten egg whites. Meanwhile, split ladyfingers. Place halves upright (flat side in) around outer sides of a 4-cup mold. When chocolate mixture is partially thickened, beat egg whites and cream of tartar until stiff. Fold into chocolate mixture; blend thoroughly. Carefully spoon into mold. Cover with clear plastic wrap. Chill for 3 to 4 hours or until set. Unmold onto a serving plate as you would any gelatin mixture. To serve, cut in six slices.

Nutritive values per serving:		
	Carbohydrates	11 grams
	Protein	7 grams
	Fat	4 grams
	Sodium	100 milligrams
	Calories	108

* Starred recipes are adapted from Katharine Middleton and Mary Abbott Hess, *The Art of Cooking for the Diabetic*. Chicago: Contem-

porary Books, 1978. © Katharine Middleton and Mary Abbott Hess. Adapted with permission of the publisher.

Food Tables

The following food tables are adapted from those distributed to patients in the Diabetes Self-Care Program. For quick calculation, the grams of carbohydrates and protein given at the beginning of each table can be used. The more exact amounts are listed for the various foods and servings. These amounts are from *Food Values of Portions Commonly Used;* other references may vary slightly, and these may be different from the values listed on a food label. A common-sense approach to measuring food and calculating grams of nutrients is what's important. A gram or two or a few calories will not make a big difference, but miscalculating by 8 or 10 grams may. Therefore, you should use these or comparable tables and, until you are adept at measuring by eye, you should use a scale and measuring cup to calculate portion sizes.

Group 1: Milk
8-oz. cup contains approximately: 12 grams carbohydrates
8 grams protein

Type of milk, serving	Calories	Carbohydrates (Grams)
Nonfat Fortified Milk		
Skim or nonfat milk, 1 cup	89	11.9
Powdered (nonfat dry, before adding liquid), 1/3 cup	84	12.2
Canned, evaporated skim milk, 1/2 cup	92	13.6
Buttermilk made from skim milk, 1 cup	88	12.4

Low-Fat Fortified Milk

	Calories	Carbohydrates (Grams)
1% fat fortified milk (add 2.5 grams fat), 1 cup	105	12.2
2% fat fortified milk (add 5 grams fat), 1 cup	125	12.2

Whole Milk

	Calories	Carbohydrates (Grams)
Whole milk (add 8 grams fat), 1 cup	150	11.5
Canned evaporated milk (add 8 grams fat), 1/2 cup	137	9.7
Buttermilk made from whole milk (add 4 grams fat), 1 cup	92	9.5
Condensed, sweet (add 5 grams fat), 1 T.	64	10.9

Yogurt (plain, unflavored)*

	Calories	Carbohydrates (Grams)
Lowfat yogurt (add 2.5 grams fat), 1 cup	122	12.6
Whole milk yogurt (add 8 grams fat), 1 cup	152	12.0

* Yogurt figures are from U.S. Department of Agriculture.
Note: 1 gram fat = 9 calories.

Group 2: VEGETABLES
One serving contains approximately: 4–7 grams carbohydrates
2 grams protein

	Calories	Carbohydrates (Grams)
Vegetables, cooked		
Asparagus, 2/3 cup	20	3.6
Bean sprouts, 1 cup	28	5.2
Beans, green, 1/2 cup	20	4.6
Beets, 1/2 cup diced	27	6.0

	Calories	Carbohydrates (Grams)
Broccoli, 2/3 cup	26	4.5
Brussels sprouts, 2/3 cup	36	6.4
Cabbage, 1/2 cup	8	1.3
Carrots, 2/3 cup	31	7.1
Cauliflower, 7/8 cup	22	4.1
Cocktail vegetable juice, 2/5 cup	21	5.0
Eggplant, 1/2 cup diced	19	4.1
Greens: cooked		
Beet, 1/2 cup	18	3.3
Chard, 3/5 cup	18	3.3
Collard, 1/2 cup	29	4.9
Dandelion, 1/2 cup	33	6.4
Kale, with stems, 3/4 cup	28	4.0
Mustard, 1/2 cup	23	4.0
Spinach, 1/2 cup	21	3.2
Turnip, 2/3 cup	19	3.3
Okra, 8–9 pods	29	6.0
Onions, 1/2 cup	29	6.5
Pepper, green, 3 1/2 oz.	18	3.8
Rutabaga, cubed, 1/2 cup	35	8.2
Sauerkraut, 2/3 cup	18	4.0
Tomato, boiled, 1/2 cup	26	5.5
Zucchini, 1/2 cup	14	3.1
Vegetables, raw		
Cabbage, shredded, 1 cup	24	5.4
Celery, diced, 1 cup	17	3.9
Chicory, 30 to 40 leaves	20	3.8
Chinese cabbage, 1 cup	16	2.6
Cucumber, 1 medium	16	3.4
Endive, 20 long leaves	20	4.1
Escarole, 4 large leaves	20	4.1
Lettuce, all kinds, 3 1/2 oz.	16	3.0
Mushrooms, 10 small/4 large	28	4.4

Parsley, 3 1/2 oz.	44	8.5
Pepper, green, 1 large shell	22	4.8
Radishes, 10 small	17	3.6
Spinach, 3 1/2 oz.	26	4.3
Tomato, 1 small	22	4.7
Watercress, 3 1/2 oz.	19	3.0

Starchy vegetables are listed in Group 4

Group 3: FRUIT
One serving contains approximately: 15–20 grams carbohydrates

Fruit, serving size	Calories	Carbohydrates (Grams)
Apple, 2 3/4″ diameter, 5 oz.	87	21.7
Apple juice, 2/3 cup, 5 oz.	75	18.5
Applesauce, unsweetened, 8 oz.	82	21.6
Apricots, dried, 1 1/2″ diameter, 6 halves, 1 oz.	92	23.0
Apricots, fresh, 4 medium, 6.5 oz.	68	17.0
Avocado, 1/3 cup cubed	80	3.0
Banana, 6″ long	85	22.2
Berries		
Blackberries, 1 cup*	84	18.6
Blueberries, 1 cup	87	21.4
Raspberries, black, 2/3 cup*	75	15.7
Raspberries, red, 1 cup*	76	18.1
Strawberries, 15 large or 1 1/2 cups*	84	18.9
Cherries, whole, 15 large	70	17.4
Cranberries, unsweetened, 1 cup*	46	10.8
Dates, pitted, whole, 3 medium*	82	21.9
Figs, dried, 2 small	82	20.7
Figs, fresh, 2 large or 3 medium	80	20.3
Fruit cocktail, unsweetened, 1 cup	74	19.4

	Calories	Carbohydrates (Grams)
Grapefruit, 4" diameter, 1 whole	82	21.6
Grapefruit juice, unsweetened, 1 cup	75	19.0
Grapes, green or red, 3/4 cup or 28 medium	80	20.7
Kumquats, 5–6 medium*	65	17.1
Mango, 2/3 cup diced or sliced	66	16.8
Melon		
Cantaloupe, 5" diameter, 1/2 melon	60	14.5
Honeydew, 10" diameter, 1/2 melon	66	15.4
Watermelon, cubed, 1 cup*	52	12.4
Nectarine, 2 medium	64	17.1
Orange, 1 medium	73	18.3
Orange juice, 3/4 cup, 6 oz.	83	19.3
Papaya, 2/3 medium or 4/5 cup mashed	78	20.0
Peach, 2 medium	76	19.4
Pear, 1/2 medium*	61	15.3
Pears, canned, unsweetened, 1 cup	80	20.7
Persimmon, native, 1/2 medium	63.5	16.7
Pineapple chunks, frozen, unsweetened, 3/8 cup	85	22.2
Pineapple, diced, 1 cup (raw)	86.6	22.8
Pineapple juice, 5 oz.	80	20.5
Pineapple, sliced, unsweetened, 2 (3 1/2" × 3/4") slices	88	22.5
Plums, raw, 2 medium	66	17.8
Prune juice, 2/5 cup	77	19.0
Prunes, unsweetened, 2 large	86	22.8
Raisins, 3 T.	87	23.1
Rhubarb, raw, cubed, 1 cup	16	3.7
Tangelos, 2 medium	78	18.4
Tangerine, 3 small	69	17.4

* High in fiber (over 1.2 grams per serving).

Group 4: STARCHES (bread, cereal, grains, starchy vegetables)
One serving contains: *Items contain:
about 11–16 grams carbohydrates   about 20 grams carbohydrates
          3 grams protein   2 grams protein

	Calories	Carbohydrates (Grams)
Bread: (Use information on labels for more exact nutrient content)		
Bagel, small, 1/2 bagel	82	15.0
Biscuit, 1 average	91	14.6
Bran muffin, 1 average	104	17.2
Bread crumbs, dried, 1/4 cup	86	16.0
Bread sticks, plain, 31/2 average	80	15.8
Bread stuffing, 1/3 cup*	87	8.2
Cinnamon raisin, 1 average slice	60	12.6
Corn bread, 1 piece	105	15.0
Corn bread stuffing, 1/4 cup	88	17.0
Corn muffin, 1 average*	130	19.0
Croutons, 1 oz.*	102	21.0
English muffin, 1/2 muffin	69	14.0
Frankfurter roll, 1 whole	108	18.9
Hamburger roll, 1 whole	89	15.9
Pita, 1/2 large or 1 small	80	14.0
Popover, 1 average	112	12.9
Pumpernickel, 1 slice	79	17.0
Roll, dinner, 1 average	75	13.4
Shake'n'Bake, plain, 3 T.	90	9.3
Tortilla, corn, white or yellow, 1 average	63	13.5
White, Italian, French, 1 average slice	60	11.5
Whole wheat, rye, 1 average slice	56	11
Crackers		
Animal crackers, 10 pieces	86	16.0
Arrowroot, 3 cookies	70	11.0

	Calories	Carbohydrates (Grams)
Escort, 4 crackers	78	10.2
Graham, 2 crackers*	54	20.6
Matzoh, 1 piece*	117	25.4
Melba toast, 5 slices	75	13.5
Oyster, 20 crackers	86	15.0
Ritz, 3 crackers	54	12.8
Rye wafers, 3 crackers	72	15.9
Saltines, 6 crackers	84	13.8
Soda, 2 crackers	61	9.9
Triscuits, 4 crackers	84	12.4
Uneeda biscuits, 4 crackers	84	14.2
Vanilla wafers, 4 cookies	68	11.0
Wheat Thins, 8 pieces	72	10.0
Zwieback, 2 pieces	62	11.8

Cereal

	Calories	Carbohydrates (Grams)
40% bran flakes, 1 cup*	106	28.2
Corn flakes, 1 cup*	83	18.9
Cream of Wheat, 1/2 cup	66	14.1
Grits, corn, cooked, 1/2 cup	61	13.4
Oatmeal, cooked, 1/2 cup	74	13.0
Puffed cereal, 1 cup	50	10.5

Grains

	Calories	Carbohydrates (Grams)
Barley, raw, 1/8 cup*	87	19.7
Cornmeal, uncooked, 2 T.	65	14.0
Cornstarch, tapioca, uncooked, 2 T.	70	17.0
Couscous, 1/2 cup	105	22.0
Flour, all-purpose, 2 1/2 T.	72	15.2
Pancake, cooked, 1 average	104	15.3
Pasta: macaroni, spaghetti, etc.		
cooked tender, 1/2 cup	80	16.0
cooked firm, 1/2 cup	105	23.0
Egg noodles, cooked, 1/2 cup*	100	18.6

Popcorn, popped (no fat added),		
1¹/2 cup	76	16.0
Rice, white, cooked, ¹/2 cup*	82	18.0
Wheat germ, 2 T.	72	9.4

Starchy Vegetables

Baked beans (with pork and		
tomato), ¹/3 cup	101	15.8
Corn on the cob, 4"-long ear	100	21.0
Corn niblets, cooked, ¹/2 cup	70	16.4
Kidney beans, cooked, ¹/3 cup	98	17.8
Lentils, dried, cooked, ¹/2 cup	79	14.5
Lentils, dried, raw, ¹/8 cup	85	30.0
Lima beans, cooked, ¹/2 cup	89	15.8
Mixed vegetables, cooked, ²/3 cup	77	16.2
Parsnips, diced, cooked, ¹/2 cup	66	14.9
Peas, green, cooked, ²/3 cup	71	12.1
Plantain, green, 5" long	119	31.2
Potato, white, without skin, 2¹/4"		
diameter*	95	21.1
Potato, white, mashed with milk		
and margarine, ¹/2 cup	94	12.3
Pumpkin, canned, 1 cup*	76	18.2
Squash,		
Acorn, baked, ¹/2 squash*	86	21.8
Hubbard, boiled, 1 cup	74	16.9
Butternut, baked, ¹/2 cup	69	17.9
Winter, baked, ¹/2 cup	63	15.4
Yam or sweet potato, baked with		
skin, ¹/2 small	70	16.0

Group 5: PROTEIN FOODS
One serving = 5 oz. unless specified otherwise

A. Lean	Calories	Fat *(in grams)*	Protein *(in grams)*
BEEF:			
Chuck steak, lean, cooked	321	14.2	45.0
Flank steak, lean only, cooked	316	10.6	51.4
Round, bottom, lean only, broiled	357	14.2	53.0
Round, top, lean only, broiled	324	7.8	58.0
Rump, lean only, pot-roasted	311	11.3	48.0
LAMB:			
Leg, lean only, roasted	263	8.5	43.1
Loin chop, lean only, cooked	278	11.0	41.9
Rib chop, lean only, cooked	293	12.4	42.9
PORK:			
Ham, fresh, lean only, cooked	334	9.6	58.0
Loin chop, lean only, cooked	374	16.9	51.7
Picnic shoulder, lean only, roasted	269	8.9	43.6
VEAL:			
Cutlet, round, lean only, cooked	415	27.4	49.6
Loin chop, lean only, cooked	310	9.9	51.2
Rib chop, lean only, cooked	322	11.9	50.3
POULTRY:			
Chicken, broiler, flesh only, broiled	204	5.7	35.7

Turkey, all classes, flesh only, roasted	285	9.2	47.3

FISH:

Clams, meat only	120	28.0	16.6
Flounder, baked	303	12.3	45.0
Salmon, Atlantic, canned	304	12.2	32.5
Sardines, canned in brine or mustard	294	18.0	28.2
Scallops, bay or sea, steamed	168	2.1	34.8
Tuna, canned in water, solids and liquid	190	1.2	42.0

DAIRY:

Cottage cheese, uncreamed, 2% fat	135	2.9	20.7
Cottage cheese, uncreamed 1% fat	108.6	1.5	18.6

B. Medium Fat

BEEF:

Chuck, ground, cooked	490	35.8	39.0
Corned, medium fat, canned	321	18.2	38.0
Ribeye steak, cooked	660	59.1	29.8

PORK:

Canadian bacon, broiled or fried	464	29.8	44.0
Loin chop, lean with some fat, cooked	535.5	33.7	38.8
Shoulder blade, lean and marbled, cooked	412	25.3	43.0

ORGAN MEATS:

Beef heart, lean, braised	268	8.5	46.9
Beef kidney, braised	378	18.0	49.5
Calf sweetbreads, braised	252	4.8	48.9
Calves' liver, fried	391	19.8	44.0

	Calories	Fat *(in grams)*	Protein *(in grams)*
DAIRY:			
Cottage cheese, creamed	159	6.3	20.1
Egg, boiled, 1 egg	78	5.5	6.2
Mozzarella, 1 oz.	79	6.1	5.4
Neufchâtel, 1 oz.	73	6.6	2.8
Parmesan, hard, 1 oz.	111	7.3	10.1
Ricotta, 1/2 cup	216	16.1	14.5

C. High Fat

	Calories	Fat *(in grams)*	Protein *(in grams)*
BEEF:			
Brisket, including fat, cooked	645	58.7	27.1
Corned, medium fat, cooked	558	45.6	34.3
Hamburger, medium fat, cooked	394	25.5	45.6
LAMB:			
Shoulder chop, including fat, cooked	510	39.0	36.9
POULTRY:			
Duck, domestic, roasted	465	35.4	34.2
Goose, flesh and skin, roasted	661	57.2	34.4
PORK:			
Spare ribs, roasted	410	33.2	20.5
MISCELLANEOUS:			
American cheese, pasteurized, processed, 1 oz.	107	8.4	6.5
Bologna, 1 slice	88	8.2	3.4
Cheddar cheese, American, 1 oz.	112	9.1	7.0

Frankfurter, cooked, 1

average	124	10.0	7.0
Peanut butter, 1 T.	86	7.2	3.9

Group 6: FATS
One serving contains: 5 grams fat
45 calories

	Serving Size	Calories
POLYUNSATURATED:		
Almonds†	6 nuts	45.0
Avocado (4" diameter)†	1/8	46.0
Margarine, soft, tub or stick*	1 tsp.	36.0
Oil, corn, cottonseed, safflower, soy, sunflower	1 tsp.	42.0
Oil, olive†	1 tsp.	41.0
Oil, Peanut†	1 tsp.	41.0
Olives†	6 med.	45.0
Peanuts, roasted with skin†	1/2 oz.	40.0
Pecans	5 halves	43.0
Walnuts	4–7 halves	49.0
SATURATED:		
Bacon, broiled or fried, crisp	1 strip	48.0
Bacon fat	1 tsp.	42.0
Butter	1 tsp.	36.0
Cream cheese	1 T.	50.0
Cream, heavy	1 T.	52.0
Cream, light	1 T.	44.0
Cream, sour	2 T.	52.0
French dressing‡	1 T.	57.0
Italian dressing‡	2 tsp.	51.0
Lard	1 tsp.	42.0
Margarine, regular stick	1 tsp.	36.0

	Serving Size	Calories
Mayonnaise‡	1 tsp.	33.0
Salad dressing, mayonnaise type	1 tsp.	45.0
Salt pork, raw	1 tsp.	36.5

* Made with corn, cottonseed, safflower, soy, or sunflower oil only.

† Fat content is primarily monounsaturated.

‡ If made with corn, cottonseed, safflower, soy, or sunflower oil can be used on fat-modified diet.

7

The Importance of Exercise

Exercise has long been recognized as an important component in diabetes therapy. Before the discovery of insulin, for example, doctors recommended exercise along with carbohydrate restriction as a means of trying to control blood glucose. And people with diabetes themselves know all too well that physical activity can have a profound effect on blood sugar because, unless properly timed with food intake, it can result in serious lowering of blood sugar. The trick is to make exercise a planned part of the treatment regimen. Fortunately, this is very much in keeping with the times; today's increased awareness of the benefits of exercise and physical fitness has resulted in an ever-growing number of people, including those with diabetes, engaging in some form of regular exercise. This is in sharp contrast to the situation only a few years ago, when very few diabetic patients engaged in vigorous exercise. People like the hockey player Bobby Clarke or tennis star Bill Talbert were considered rare exceptions because they were so physically active despite their diabetes.

Participants in the Diabetes Self-Care Program are urged to exercise daily; the duration and intensity vary from person to person. Before embarking on an exercise program, you should understand the effects of physical activity on insulin and blood sugar. As in so many other facets of life, you must be more attuned to your body than the nondiabetic when undertaking an exercise program. Also, since diabetes increases the risk of heart disease, you should not begin an exercise program without a doctor's approval. For most adults, this will mean undergoing a physical examination, including an exercise tolerance test, to help determine the safe level of physical activity.

BENEFITS OF EXERCISE

The person with diabetes derives many of the same benefits from exercise as nondiabetic people. These include:

• *Cardiovascular conditioning.* Exercise helps the heart and lungs work more efficiently. A well-conditioned heart pumps more blood with each beat, thus reducing the number of beats, or contractions, required to circulate the blood. This means that more oxygen-rich blood can be circulated with less strain on the heart. In addition, well-conditioned muscles—including the heart—extract more oxygen from the blood, again reducing the workload on the heart. These effects of cardiovascular conditioning are particularly important for people with diabetes because of their increased risk of coronary artery disease and heart attacks.

• *Possible lowering of high blood pressure.* Studies have found that some people with hypertension experience a moderate lowering of their blood pressure after beginning a regular exercise program. In people with mild hypertension, this may be adequate to bring blood pressure into the normal zone, another important effect for diabetic patients because hypertension compounds the risk of heart disease. How exercise may lower blood pressure is unknown, although most experts believe it is probably a combination of factors, including increased cardiovascular efficiency, weight loss, and reduced stress.

• *Improved insulin sensitivity.* Studies have found that regular exercise increases the ability of the cells to use insulin, which explains why diabetic patients who exercise regularly often are able to reduce their insulin dosage.

• *Improved weight control.* Weight loss during exercise conditioning is common, even among people who eat more than they did previously. Not only does the physical activity burn calories, it also helps the body's natural appetite control to function better. Exercise is particularly important for people on a weight-loss diet because it helps overcome the metabolic slowdown that results from a large weight reduction. It also promotes the breakdown of fat stores, and since fatty tissue increases insulin resistance, this can help promote insulin uptake. Many overweight people with type 2 diabetes, for example, can control their disease with a regimen of weight loss and exercise.

• *Lowering of cholesterol and other lipids.* People who exercise regularly tend to have lower levels of blood cholesterol and triglycerides. In addition, regular exercise appears to increase the level of HDL cholesterol, the type that is considered protective against heart disease. Cholesterol is a fatty substance, and since fat and water, the major component of blood, do not mix, cholesterol must be attached to another substance to circulate through the body. This substance is a lipoprotein (which means lipid-carrying protein). There are several types of lipoproteins. The largest are the high-density lipoproteins, and they appear to carry cholesterol away from the cells. In contrast, the smaller, low-density lipoproteins, or LDL cholesterol, carry cholesterol to the cells. The very low-density lipoproteins, or VLDL, carry mostly triglycerides, lipids that are often at elevated levels in people with diabetes.

The higher the level of HDL cholesterol in relationship to LDL the better. Elevated cholesterol is thought to be a major factor in the development of atherosclerosis, the buildup of fatty deposits along the artery walls. As atherosclerosis progresses, it causes a narrowing of the coronary arteries, which reduces the blood supply to the heart muscle. Very often a coronary artery that is diseased by atherosclerosis will become completely blocked, either by a blood clot (coronary thrombus) or by the fatty plaque itself. This is the major cause of heart attacks and death in this country. Most people living in industrialized societies, including Americans, have a higher level of blood cholesterol than that seen in population groups from rural, less-developed countries. A high-fat diet, sedentary lifestyle, and stress all are thought to be factors contributing to elevated cholesterol. Since the diet recommended for those with diabetes tends to be higher in fat and lower in carbohydrates than that recommended for the nondiabetic population, you should take whatever measures you can to control cholesterol and other blood lipids. Thus exercise is particularly important for the diabetic patient who wants to promote cardiovascular health. (For a more detailed discussion, see Chapter 12.)

• *Stress reduction.* People who exercise regularly are better able to cope with stress than their more sedentary counterparts. Most of us know avid runners who speak (often at boring length) about the sense of well-being achieved from jogging or running. They talk about a runner's high, and many seem to be addicted to their daily workout; if they miss a day or two of exercise, they feel on edge and jittery, sensations akin to withdrawal symptoms. Biochemical analyses of the blood of people who exercise have found that they produce high levels of endorphins, substances that are produced in the brain and mimic the effects of morphine. These natural chemicals produce a feeling of euphoria and blunt pain, explaining why many marathoners and competitive athletes can finish a race or game even though they have suffered an injury that would normally be very painful. Elevated levels of endorphins can help overcome stress and promote relaxation and a feeling of emotional well-being. Since stress is increasingly linked to a growing list of diseases, most doctors agree that positive steps to reduce stress are beneficial to health. In any event, the fact that exercise simply makes you feel better would seem to justify the effort.

• *Improved blood vessel and muscle tone.* Increased use improves the tone of both skeletal and vascular muscles. Conditioned muscles that are exercised regularly require increased amounts of glycogen, the stored form of blood glucose. The more glycogen that is stored in the muscles and liver, the better able a person is to counter episodes of low blood sugar.

Conditioned athletes have a higher ratio of muscle to body fat than do nonexercisers, explaining why many athletes look trim even though they may weigh more than more sedentary people. Improved tone of vascular muscles helps improve circulation, an important benefit for diabetic patients, who have an increased risk of circulatory problems.

• *Reduced risk of blood clotting.* Recent studies at Duke Medical Center and several other major medical institutions have found that regular exercise may affect the body's ability to produce or dissolve blood clots. The formation of tiny clots in the blood vessels is thought to be a possible initiating factor in atherosclerosis. These clots form at the sites of injury along the artery walls. The initial causes of the injuries are unknown; researchers have suggested they may be due to increased turbulence of high blood pressure, allergic responses, viruses, or other, unknown circumstances. Platelets, the minute corpuscles in the blood that are instrumental in the clotting process, clump at the site of these injuries, releasing chemicals that constrict the blood vessels even more. Fatty deposits accumulate, setting in motion the atherosclerotic process. Regular exercise is believed to increase the body's ability to dissolve these clots; it also may reduce the stickiness of platelets, thus lowering their clumping at the site of arterial injury.

Effects of Exercise on Diabetes

During exercise, the body requires more fuel to maintain the increased activity. When a nondiabetic person exercises, blood glucose levels remain stable; the glucose burned by the working muscles is constantly replaced by available stores from digested food and also from the conversion of stored glycogen into glucose. The pancreas excretes very little insulin during exercise because the increased activity is burning the excess sugar. To meet the fuel needs of muscles during prolonged exercise, the liver increases the amount of available glucose by converting glycogen to sugar. If this is insufficient, as might be the case during vigorous exercise lasting more than twenty minutes, the body begins breaking down some of its stored fat and converting it to glucose. If the exercise continues long enough, for example, a long-distance race or a few hours of cross-country skiing, the liver will begin producing glucose from protein. These changes take place largely because of hormonal activity during exercise; namely, the excretion of antiinsulin hormones such as glucagon, cortisol, ACTH (growth hormone), and catecholamines.

These metabolic processes are somewhat different in the diabetic patient. The person with diabetes, of course, does not have a functioning pancreas to reduce the amount of available insulin during exercise; instead, the amount of insulin in the body will depend on the time, dose, and type of insulin injection. For example, if you exercise when blood glucose is on the high side, it generally will fall rather than remain stable, as is the case with the nondiabetic person. Thus, you can use exercise to lower moderately elevated blood sugar without having to take extra insulin. But extremes should be avoided; if blood sugar is very high—say, 300 mg/dl or more—exercise may send it even higher. Studies by Dr. Philip Felig and his colleagues at the Yale University School of Medicine have found that exercise in people with poorly controlled diabetes, whose blood sugar is very high, results in an exaggerated increase in antiinsulin hormones, which leads to increased glucose production. In addition, problems may occur if exercise is undertaken when blood sugar is on the low end of the scale, especially if it will coincide with an insulin peak. In such cases, blood sugar may be dangerously depleted, resulting in hypoglycemia. To further complicate matters, the response to exercise is not always predictable. A number of factors, including such things as site of injection, level of physical fitness, and regularity of exercise, can alter the effect on blood sugar. Obviously, you must plan your exercise activities more carefully than the nondiabetic person.

TYPES OF EXERCISE

In general, there are three types of exercise: aerobic, anaerobic, and stretching. Aerobic, or dynamic, exercise is any activity that involves prolonged, repetitive use of large muscles, thus increasing the body's need for oxygen. Examples of aerobic exercise include brisk walking, jogging, swimming, cycling, rope skipping, and cross-country skiing. This type of exercise promotes cardiovascular fitness and efficiency.

Anaerobic, or static, exercise are those activities in which the energy demands of the muscles are supplied without an increased need for oxygen. They are of short duration and involve such activities as sprinting, weight-lifting, or downhill skiing. This type of exercise conditions, strengthens, and tones muscles, but does not improve cardiovascular fitness. Weight-lifting and other anaerobic exercises generally are not recommended for people with high blood pressure or for those who suffer retinal hemorrhages because such activities may worsen these conditions.

Stretching exercises are designed to strengthen ligaments and tendons and to promote greater flexibility. They include such activities as yoga and calisthenics. Each exercise session should be preceded and followed by five to ten minutes of warm-up and cool-down stretching exercises. These will help prevent injuries and problems such as muscle cramps.

Exercise programs for diabetic patients are built around aerobic exercises. To promote cardiovascular conditioning and gain the maximum benefit from physical activity, the exercise session must be long and hard enough to increase the heart rate (the number of beats per minute) into the prescribed training or conditioning range. In addition, the exercise must be performed regularly, at least three or four times a week. Patients in the Diabetes Self-Care Program are urged to exercise daily if at all possible, or at least three or four times a week. This means that exercise becomes a regular, planned part of the therapeutic regimen. In addition to achieving better blood glucose control, the diabetic patient who exercises regularly will also improve cardiovascular fitness.

HOW TO GET STARTED

First check with your doctor. Depending on your age and the presence of other risk factors, an exercise tolerance test may be recommended to develop a safe exercise prescription. This test, which provides a direct means of measuring the heart's work capacity, involves exercising, either on a treadmill or exercise bicycle, while undergoing continuous electrocardiographic monitoring. Electrodes from the electrocardiogram machine are attached to specific places on your chest, and a doctor or technician will observe the printout for changes in heart rhythm and other abnormalities. Blood pressure also will be monitored before, during, and after the test; in some instances, lung function and certain other cardiovascular responses may be measured as well.

The test usually is administered in a doctor's office, clinic, or hospital outpatient department. It involves little risk, but personnel trained in administering the test and handling any emergency that might arise should supervise it. When undergoing an exercise test, wear loose, comfortable exercise clothing and sneakers or running shoes. The exercise will be performed at increasing intensity until your heart rate reaches a predetermined level or until you are too tired to continue. The test may be stopped if abnormal heart rhythms or other symptoms occur or if you appear to be overly anxious. Using the information from an exercise test, a doctor or other trained health professional, such as an exercise physiologist, can determine your heart's present work capacity and design an exercise prescription to increase cardiovascular fitness. In the absence of a specific exercise prescription, you can use the following guidelines to design an individual conditioning program.

When you undertake an exercise program, especially if you have been rather sedentary up to this point, there is one other cardinal rule: *start slowly and build up gradually.* Far too many people make the mistake of thinking they can get in shape in a few days, and they try to do too much too fast. This is self-defeating because it increases the chance of injury and also can be very discouraging when the hoped-for results are not achieved immediately. Remember, most people who take up exercise have years of sedentary living behind them; they also have the rest of their lives to get back in shape. How long this takes depends on age, overall physical condition, and the presence of medical problems. As Self-Care exercise physiologists note, even healthy professional athletes require months of training before beginning a new season; it seems unrealistic to expect that a formerly sedentary person can achieve fitness in less time than that required by a pro. Overdoing in the beginning not only can raise havoc with joints and muscles, it also can upset your blood glucose control.

Many people also make the mistake of assuming that because they have encountered problems in the past, they should not attempt exercise conditioning. Almost everyone, including amputees and people with severely limiting heart disease, can benefit from an exercise program. For people with special medical problems, such as heart disease or serious circulatory or orthopedic disorders, extra attention should be paid to the design of the program. These people also may want to start by exercising in a controlled setting, such as an exercise clinic or special class at the YMCA, at least in the beginning.

In designing an exercise program, select activities that are enjoyable, accessible, and safe. You may love swimming, which is an excellent aerobic exercise. But if you have access to a pool for only a couple of months out of the year, it obviously is not the best choice for a year-round exercise program. Walking is an ideal choice for most people. It is inexpensive—the only equipment required is a good, properly fitted pair of shoes—and does not require special skills. Walking at a brisk pace can provide the desired cardiovascular conditioning without causing the harm to weight-bearing joints that is so often incurred in jogging. In fact, orthopedic considerations are paramount in designing an exercise-conditioning program, since more exercisers are sidelined by joint, tendon, or muscle injuries than any other health factor.

Jogging and running are also popular choices for an exercise program. The cadence of jogging, although not much faster than a brisk walk, provides a more vigorous cardiovascular workout. By the same token, the up-and-down motion also means more potential orthopedic damage, especially among people who are overweight and out of condition. Therefore, if you are just embarking on an exercise program, it is a good idea to start with walking, gradually increasing the distance and speed, and if a more vigorous exercise is desired, to slowly incorporate jogging into the walking program.

Other excellent conditioning exercises include cycling, either on a stationary bicycle or ergometer, or a regular bicycle; aerobic dancing (if your joints can tolerate the activity); ice or roller skating, and walking in water (particularly good for people with orthopedic problems who have access to a level, shallow pool). Games, such as tennis, handball, squash, and volleyball, may provide good conditioning exercise if played vigorously and regularly. For those who are in good physical condition and have their diabetes under good control, sports requiring considerable endurance, such as cross-country skiing, hiking, rowing, or even running a marathon, are feasible.

THE BASICS OF EXERCISE CONDITIONING

Exercise conditioning depends on intensity, frequency, and duration of the training activity. Intensity is determined by the training heart rate. For people with no cardiovascular problems, this is generally defined as a heart rate (beats per minute) that is 70 to 80 percent of the maximum attainable rate. To calculate the maximum heart rate, subtract your age from 220; this will be within 12 beats per minute (plus or minus) of what your heart is capable of. (For example, if you are 30 years old, your safe maximum heart rate would be 190 beats per minute, plus or minus 12, or a range of 178 to 202.) Your training range would be 70 to 80 percent of that. (Some cardiovascular conditioning programs recommend a range of 70 to 85 percent, but exercise physiologists at the Diabetes Self-Care Program set the recommended upper limit at 80 percent.) Thus, the recommended training range for a 30-year-old with no compromising heart problems would be 133 to 152 beats per minute.

To determine whether the conditioning heart rate has been attained, you must learn to take your own pulse. This is easily done and requires only a watch with a second hand. There are a number of places where you can count your pulse: you usually can find it easily by tipping your hand back and pressing a finger on your wrist, just above the palm. You also can find the pulse by pressing a finger against the artery located in the temple, or on the side of the neck, below the ear. Practice finding pulse points and then counting the pulses (which correspond to heartbeats). Count the beats for ten seconds and then multiply by six to get the heart rate per minute. Do this before starting to exercise and again immediately after stopping. (You also may want to take your pulse after exercising for a few minutes to make sure you are in your training range.) With a bit of practice, you should have no trouble taking your pulse.

In the beginning, it is not necessary to push yourself into your target training range, especially if you are out of condition. It is more important to get the muscles and body used to exercising—something that may take a few weeks to accomplish. With each session, you can strive for a progressively higher heart rate until you reach your training range.

Frequency is as important as intensity in beginning an exercise conditioning program. For conditioning to have its desired effect, the exercise must be performed at least three times a week, preferably on alternating days. For those with diabetes, daily sessions of increasing intensity and duration are generally preferable to a thrice-weekly schedule. This will strengthen the muscles and skeletal system and also provide the consistency needed to help control blood glucose.

Duration, the third factor, depends on physical condition. In general, twenty to thirty minutes of exercise in the target heart-rate zone is the minimum needed for cardiovascular conditioning. At the outset, you may feel tired after only a few minutes of vigorous exercise. If this is the case, decrease the intensity (walk or cycle at a slower pace, for example). You may start by walking a mile in twenty minutes, and gradually speed this up until you can walk a mile in fifteen minutes with your heart rate in the training range for most of that time. Then, as you become more fit and your body is more accustomed to the activity, you can increase the distance covered until you can walk two miles in thirty minutes with your heart in the training range. Again, once this goal has been achieved, strive for a brisker pace, say two miles in twenty-six minutes, and at the same time extend the distance until you are walking thirty to forty minutes with your heart rate in the training range. As you become more physically fit, you will find that you have to walk faster and further to stay in your training range. This means that you are achieving a basic objective: your heart is able to work more efficiently with less effort.

Of course, you should take extra precautions. As noted earlier, timing of the exercise is important. Measure blood glucose before and immediately after a workout and again an hour later. Keep a careful record of your glucose measurements as well as the length of the exercise session. As the amount of exercise is increased, there should be a greater lowering of blood glucose. As Dr. Peterson explains: "When you are in poor physical condition, a thirty-minute exercise session may lower your blood glucose only 10 mg/dl. As you achieve greater physical fitness, the glucose-lowering effect will increase because the muscles will be storing more glycogen. It is not unusual for a well-conditioned person with diabetes to have blood glucose fall 50 or 60 mg/dl during thirty minutes of vigorous exercise. In addition, the glucose may continue to fall at a slower rate for up to five hours after the exercise.

"After you know how much of an effect you consistently get from an exercise session, you can learn to use exercise in much the same way as you use Regular insulin to produce a fast lowering of blood glucose." Some diabetic patients find they can use exercise to substitute for some of their insulin.

The blood sugar level at the start of an exercise session is the key factor in determining whether a food supplement should be taken before beginning. In general, if blood sugar is 75 mg/dl or lower, a supplement of fruit juice will be needed. The amount depends on the duration and intensity of exercise and individual response to it. The best way to determine this is to measure your blood sugar and if it is above 75 mg/dl, exercise for ten minutes, then measure it again, noting any decrease. Take a third measurement an hour later. If the blood sugar drops too low, eat enough carbohydrates (a calibrated amount of milk, fruit juice, or other source of simple sugar) to produce the needed glucose. By doing this over a period of several days with increasing amounts of exercise, you can gauge how your body is likely to respond to the exercise.

During a prolonged session, such as a long run or a competitive event, you should break for a glucose measurement. If it is inconvenient to carry a glucose meter, just using the reagent strips will be sufficient. Of course, you should also carry an appropriate snack. Even if your diabetes is under good control, you should strive to maintain blood sugar that is in the normal range during an exercise session and also to take precautions to ensure that it does not fall further after the workout. "If your starting blood glucose is in the normal or low-normal range, take a small amount of fruit juice or other source of simple sugar before exercising," Dr. Peterson advises. "Take a similar additional amount every ten minutes or so during the exercise session. You should then end the exercise with a normal blood sugar, which should be tested again an hour later."

OTHER FACTORS TO BE CONSIDERED

Although glucose control may be the most important factor affecting your response to exercise, there are a number of other considerations. These include:

• *Site of insulin injection.* Studies have found that exercise of an injection site may increase the rate at which insulin is absorbed. For example, if a jogger uses the thigh as an injection site, the leg exercise can speed up the rate at which the insulin will be absorbed by 50 to 135 percent, according to studies by Dr. Felig and his Yale colleagues. Obviously, this accelerated insulin absorption can result in an unexpected lowering of blood glucose. The Yale researchers found, however, that there was no increased absorption if the insulin was injected into an unexercised extremity, such as the arm, and that it was actually slowed when an abdominal site was used. Therefore, doctors advise avoiding using areas of the body that will be exercised as injection sites if you plan a subsequent workout.

• *Timing of exercise to avoid insulin peak.* Timing of exercise is important in avoiding excessive lowering of blood sugar. Insulin injections are planned to match peak effectiveness with rises in blood sugar after eating. If you know that your insulin is going to peak shortly after lunch, for example, you should either avoid exercising at this time or lower your insulin and use the exercise to cover the food intake. Such adjustments take practice and are not always predictable. In the beginning, you should master maintaining normal blood glucose while exercising by increasing carbohydrate intake. Once you have learned this, you can experiment with adjusting or lowering insulin dosage.

SUMMING UP

Exercise is an important component in the effective treatment of diabetes. It also can lead to problems of blood sugar that is too low or too high if it is not timed correctly. In general, complications can be avoided by increasing carbohydrate intake before a workout and not exercising when insulin action is peaking. Regular exercise also may enable the person with type 1 diabetes to reduce total insulin intake or increase insulin sensitivity in the type 2 diabetes patient. Before you embark on a program of exercise training, consult a physician. A specific exercise prescription may be recommended; if not, you may follow the guidelines offered in this chapter to design your own program. In any event, frequent self-monitoring of blood sugar both before and after exercise is important, especially in the beginning, until you know how your body is likely to respond to a given amount of physical activity. If properly approached, exercise conditioning can reward you with the same benefits enjoyed by the general population: increased cardiovascular fitness and lowered heart risk factors, better weight control, and an enhanced sense of well-being. In addition, you can expect to achieve improved blood glucose control.

8

Using an Insulin Pump

In the last few years, an increasing number of people with type 1 diabetes have switched to a portable, computerized pump to administer their insulin. This system, known as continuous subcutaneous insulin infusion or, more commonly, an insulin pump, replaces the syringe injections administered by type 1 and other patients with insulin-dependent diabetes. The pump device constantly delivers small amounts of insulin to cover basal needs and larger doses (boluses) before meals or when extra insulin is needed.

Although the first experiments with continuous insulin infusion were conducted in 1934, it has only been in the last decade that portable insulin pumps, which the patient can wear continually, have been developed. There are now a number of different devices available, but all operate on the same general principle. The pump itself is a small boxlike device that contains a syringelike reservoir to hold a day's supply of insulin and a battery and miniature electronic equipment. The insulin reservoir is attached to tubing and a small needle that is inserted into subcutaneous tissue at a convenient injection site, such as the abdomen, thigh, or arm. The devices, which range in size from a package the size of a deck of cards to that of a small tape recorder, can be carried in a pocket or attached to a belt.

Studies comparing the glucose control achieved by patients using the traditional insulin injections with that of people on insulin pumps have found that the pump patients come closer to achieving normal blood sugar levels. Some studies have also found a reduction in long-term complications, such as neuropathy, among patients on the pump, and some doctors now recommend it for patients who have complications or are at high risk of developing them. This does not mean, however, that the pump is appropriate for all patients. People who have a regular lifestyle and are able to keep their disease under good control with insulin injections may not have any need to change. Young children may not be good candidates for an insulin pump; the same is true of people who are self-conscious about wearing an external device. People with failing eyesight may have trouble caring for the pump. Some researchers have found that pump therapy may not be suitable for the patient with brittle diabetes who has wide, unpredictable swings in blood glucose levels or those who are prone to severe or rapid episodes of hypoglycemia.

The pump is often ideal for patients who lead somewhat irregular lifestyles but are highly motivated to achieve better diabetes control. This might include people whose jobs entail irregular hours or who find they are often too busy or engrossed in other activities to stop and figure out an insulin dose. It is also ideal for people who travel a lot because it can be programmed to accommodate changes in time zones. But even though the pump can be programmed to administer insulin at specific times, careful self-monitoring, including measuring blood glucose, is still required.

"We don't recommend the pump for anyone who has not mastered multiple insulin injections to normalize blood sugar," says Dr. Jovanovic. "Once this has been achieved, most people who want to try an insulin pump can learn how to use one, but it does require time and effort. In the beginning, using a pump is like being newly diagnosed as having diabetes. Just as it takes time for a newly diagnosed patient to learn about injections, diet, and other aspects of diabetes management, it takes time to become familiar with the pump."

Although an insulin pump may eventually make blood glucose control easier to achieve, it does not eliminate the need to practice the Self-Care principles of good management. For example, patients still must practice self-monitoring of their blood glucose and keep careful day-to-day charts or diaries (see Chapter 4). "At first, extra time must be spent both in physically caring for the pump itself and in analyzing what to do in certain situations," Dr. Jovanovic cautions. "As the wearer becomes more adept in using the system, much less time is required."

There are also new emotional adjustments that must be made. Patients who have switched from injections to the pump often describe being afraid to try something new. This is an understandable response, as Dr. Jovanovic explains: "These patients have learned how to control their diabetes with varying degrees of success using insulin injections. They know how to handle problems and what to do if an emergency arises. Now they are suddenly faced with a new insulin-delivery system and new problems. Many patients are frightened at the prospect of a battery failure or the pump becoming disconnected while they are sleeping. Couples often are hesitant to have sex for fear that something will happen to the pump and they may be embarrassed to ask a doctor how to manage these details. Pump failure can be a serious problem, especially for a pregnant woman. None of the problems are insurmountable, but it does mean adapting to life with a new appendage, which may be difficult. Some people may resent having a visible reminder of their diabetes or having to explain it to others. There are frustrations of learning how to use a new system, and until this is mastered, it may not seem worth the cost and effort. Even so, most people who make the necessary adjustments usually prefer it and do not go back to conventional therapy."

Once mastered, the pump allows for an even greater degree of flexibility in day-to-day activities. Some of the advantages were summed up at a Self-Care course for physicians and other health professionals by a former program patient. The patient, a young man named Thomas, explains that the pump has completely changed his life: "I teach aerobic dancing, and most of my classes are at night. Before I went on the pump, my erratic schedule made it very difficult to control my blood sugar. Since my job involves very vigorous exercise until about 10 P.M., my injection schedule was always out of kilter with my life. I would sometimes sleep through my scheduled morning injection, which would mess up the entire day. Now I can program my pump to reduce the insulin infusion when I am exercising and to increase it while I'm asleep. For the first time in years, my blood sugar is under good control and I can get a full night's sleep."

SWITCHING TO PUMP THERAPY

Close medical supervision is important in making the switch to an insulin pump. Self-Care physicians suggest that this be a team effort, which, ideally, would include the patient, physician, nurse specialist or diabetes educator, dietician, and exercise physiologist. You can make the switch either as an inpatient in the hospital or as an outpatient in a doctor's office, clinic, or hospital department. The inpatient setting has several advantages, including the security of twenty-four-hour medical assistance while you are learning and adjusting to the new system. This also allows time to test the machine for any mechanical problems.

If you switch as an outpatient, you should receive careful instructions in using the pump before you go home, and you should have a phone number where you can reach a doctor at any time should problems occur. A few days may be required to fine-tune the insulin dosage, especially if a long-acting insulin, such as Ultralente, has been used, because it may take the body a few days to clear itself of the remnants of this insulin.

Initially you must take a 3 A.M. blood sugar measurement because this will determine the basal insulin need. As in conventional therapy, the total insulin dosage is divided between basal requirements and bolus doses, the amount needed to cover food and other special circumstances, which is comparable to the Regular insulin used in conventional therapy. The basal insulin should maintain blood glucose at a constant level; this is the insulin that is constantly infused in small amounts.

In pump therapy, only Regular insulin is used. The total dosage is calculated in much the same manner as in conventional therapy (see page 55); for most people this means 0.6 units of insulin per kilogram of body weight per twenty-four hours. (Remember, insulin needs rise during pregnancy, periods of infection or emotional stress, decreased physical activity, the premenstrual week, puberty, and when certain medications, such as diuretics and steroids, are being used.) Therefore, in calculating the total insulin dosage for a 132-pound, or 60-kilogram, person, we can use the same formula as for conventional therapy:

$$60 \times 0.6 = 36 \text{ units of insulin}$$

Initially, this total dosage is divided equally between basal and bolus doses. Therefore, this 60-kilogram patient would allocate 18 units for basal infusion and the remaining 18 units to cover meals. The hourly basal infusion rate can be obtained by dividing the total (18 units in this case) by 24, which for this patient would be 0.75 units per hour.

The bolus doses are calculated according to the carbohydrate content of a meal (see Chapter 6), although the precise doses are determined by individual responses and needs. The amount of insulin given before breakfast may have to be slightly higher, even though less food is consumed, because many people tend to be insulin-resistant in the morning. As a rule of thumb, Dr. Jovanovic starts by giving 1.5 units of insulin for every 10 grams of carbohydrates consumed at breakfast and 1 unit for every 10 grams consumed at lunch and dinner. These figures are average and represent a starting point. They may be adjusted up or down according to blood glucose levels.

To illustrate how this would work in practice, we can go through a day's food intake for the hypothetical 60-kilogram patient. Assuming that this person wants to maintain present weight and distributes the day's food intake as outlined in Chapter 6, he or she would use the following table to calculate bolus doses. You will recall that the weight-maintenance allowance for a normally active adult is about 25 calories per kilogram, or a total of 1,500 for this person. In keeping with Self-Care dietary recommendations, 40 percent of this would be consumed in the form of carbohydrates, and since each gram of carbohydrates contains 4 calories, the total carbohydrate allowance would be 150 grams per day. Let's assume that this patient regularly has three meals and four snacks a day, and that he or she wants to continue on this schedule. If we further assume that 1.5 units of insulin will cover about 10 grams of carbohydrates at breakfast and that 1 unit will be needed for every 10 grams throughout the day, we would end up with the following bolus doses:

Meal or snack	% of day's calories	Grams of carbohydrates	Bolus dose (units of insulin)
Breakfast	10	15.0	2.25
Snack	5	7.5	0.75
Lunch	30	45.0	4.50
Snack	10	15.0	1.50
Dinner	30	45.0	4.50
Snack	5	7.5	0.75
Before bed	10	15.0	1.50

Generally, midmorning and midafternoon snacks are not required by patients using an insulin pump. Let's assume that this patient would like to cut out the midmorning and midafternoon snacks, adding the extra calories to lunch and dinner, and to have a single before-bed snack. The bolus doses would then become:

Meal or snack	% of day's calories	Grams of carbohydrates	Bolus dose (units of insulin)
Breakfast	10	15.0	2.50
Lunch	35	52.5	5.25
Dinner	40	60.0	6.00
Before bed	15	22.5	2.25

To fine-tune the bolus doses, blood sugar should be measured before and an hour after each meal. If it is too high before meals, this may mean that the basal insulin should be increased; if it is low, the basal insulin may have to be decreased. If blood sugar is too high after the meals (140 mg/dl), insulin should be increased by about 1 unit for every 25 mg/dl over 140 (check this). If it is low, insulin should be decreased.

In addition, some people may need to adjust the basal rate at certain times during the day. Basal insulin needs may increase at times when the body is insulin-resistant; for example, from 4 to 7 A.M. If the morning fasting blood glucose is consistently high, an increase in basal insulin during these hours may be needed. This can be calculated as follows:

• Check blood glucose at 3 A.M. and 7 A.M. (Both checks are mandatory.)

• If the 3 A.M. blood glucose is consistently 70 mg/dl or lower, decrease the basal rate by 0.03 units of insulin.

• If the 3 A.M. glucose is 70 to 100 mg/dl, leave the basal rate unchanged.

• If the 3 A.M. glucose is 100 mg/dl or greater, increase the basal rate by 0.03 units of insulin.

After the 3 A.M. glucose value has been stabilized at 70 to 100 mg/dl, the necessary adjustment can be made in the basal rate between 4 and 7 A.M. To do this, subtract the 3 A.M. value from the 7 A.M. measurement. (For example, assume that the 3 A.M. blood glucose is 100 mg/ dl and at 7 A.M. it has risen to 190 mg/dl. Subtracting 100 from 190 gives you 90 as the key figure.) Divide the difference (in this case 90) by 30, which will give you 3. Now multiply this by 0.03 units of insulin, which gives 1.44 units per hour or a total of 4.32 additional units to be infused between 4 and 7 A.M. The insulin pump should be programmed to add this amount during the predawn hours.

As a rule, the insulin requirement will go up in the first few days of pump therapy as insulin from conventional therapy is eliminated from the body. The requirement generally stabilizes over the next week or so, and then may decline after ten to fourteen days on the pump. "The decline may be particularly significant in patients whose glucose control was poor before going on the pump," Dr. Jovanovic cautions. "Therefore it is important to be alert for any decreasing insulin requirements so that hypoglycemia can be avoided." After the first two weeks, insulin requirements tend to remain fairly constant, although dosages may need to be recalculated to accommodate periods of stress, illness, weight gain, diet changes, and other conditions that affect insulin needs.

In the beginning, Dr. Jovanovic urges patients to adhere closely to set meal patterns if possible. "Increased flexibility in meal patterns and timing can be achieved after the initial dosages are determined and you become more skilled in pump therapy," she says. "But until you are stabilized on an insulin regimen and are comfortable in experimenting with the pump, we urge patients to keep diet and timing constant." After the dosages have been established and patients become familiar with modifying them, "Many pump wearers find they can delay or even skip meals or snacks without encountering low blood sugar," Dr. Jovanovic comments. However, if a meal is delayed, the bolus also must be postponed; by the same token, if a meal is skipped, the bolus also should be eliminated. "Patients should not skip the bedtime snack, however," Dr. Jovanovic warns, "because the risk of nighttime hypoglycemia is greater if you go to bed in a fasting state."

Self-Care physicians and dietitians urge their pump patients not to be afraid to experiment once they become comfortable with their new insulin delivery system. "Using the pump makes it much easier to determine the precise dose of insulin needed for a specific amount of food," Dr. Jovanovic says. To find out the effect of a slice of bread or piece of cheese, for example, simply measure your blood sugar before eating the item and again an hour later. The change in blood sugar will tell you how much insulin is needed to cover that particular amount of food. As a rule, 1 unit of insulin covers about 8 to 10 grams of carbohydrates; 10 grams of carbohydrates will raise the blood sugar about 30 mg/dl.

"Although more dietary freedom can be gained by using an insulin pump, it's important to remember that it is not a panacea," says nutritionist Joan Choppin. "Good meal planning remains a cornerstone in diabetes management, and a balanced diet is just as important for patients on an insulin pump as it is for those using conventional therapy." Choppin also cautions that many people tend to gain weight when they first go on the pump, even though their diet may stay the same. This is attributed to improved glucose control. Nutritionists or dietitians working with the patient should be aware of this possibility and keep it in mind when calculating the total number of calories.

EXERCISE AND THE PUMP

Exercise remains an integral part of diabetes therapy for pump wearers (see Chapter 7). Some of the same guidelines for insulin and exercise that apply to conventional therapy can be applied to pump patients. Prolonged vigorous exercise reduces the need for insulin or increases the need for food to avoid hypoglycemia. The best way to determine the effect of exercise is to measure blood sugar before and after a workout; if blood sugar falls to 70 mg/dl or lower, this is a sign that you should eat before exercising.

In general, exercise of short duration—for example, walking or jogging a mile—usually has little effect on basal insulin requirements. But if you exercise within two or three hours of a premeal bolus, you should reduce that amount of insulin or eat extra food. More prolonged exercise—a thirty-minute jogging session, a vigorous game of tennis, or a long, brisk walk—may require a reduction in basal insulin an hour before the exercise or consumption of extra food immediately before the activity. Long-term exercise conditioning or training may result in an overall reduction in basal insulin requirements; to determine this, you should monitor blood glucose regularly and keep a daily diary.

The pump can be worn during most exercise activities if it is well secured and will not get wet. However, some people feel more comfortable exercising with the pump disconnected. If you do so, enough insulin should be bolused to cover the basal rate during the time the pump is disconnected (see Temporary Disconnects, page 148). The duration and intensity of the exercise should be taken into consideration in calculating the disconnect bolus; if a two-hour run is planned, a lowered amount of basal insulin probably will suffice. At any rate, no more than the basal rate for four hours should be infused.

If the catheter is to be left in place while the pump is disconnected, it should be capped with a sterile top and taped securely to the skin until the exercise is completed and the pump is reattached. The insulin reservoir also should be covered with a sterile cap.

CARING FOR AN INSULIN PUMP

The pump is a machine and, like all machines, it requires preventive maintenance. All pumps are powered by batteries; some of these batteries need replacing or recharging every day or two, while some of the newer pumps have batteries that last for two or more months. In selecting a pump, you should check several factors. Does it have an alarm system, and if so, what will trigger it? Some pumps sound an alarm when the battery is low, the insulin reservoir is empty, for any electronic or mechanical fault, and when the pump action is suspended or malfunctioning. The type of infusion program is also important. All provide continuous infusion of basal insulin, but some can be programmed to automatically increase or decrease this at specific times. Most require manual or electronic meal boluses, although some provide preprogrammed bolus administration. Some hold only a day's supply of insulin; others have a reservoir capacity of several days.

Before beginning pump therapy, a patient should be thoroughly familiar with the system and its features. Most pump manufacturers have representatives who meet with the patient and medical team that will supervise its use. These representatives can provide literature and answer questions about everything from problem solving to maintenance. Some of those who meet with Self-Care classes are diabetic patients who use insulin pumps themselves and can answer all sorts of practical questions. For example, one of these representatives, a young woman, was particularly helpful in showing Connie how the pump can be concealed in hidden pockets that she has sewn into her suit jackets and dresses.

In addition to the actual insulin pump, the needed supplies include Betadine and alcohol swabs, an insulin syringe, insulin (Regular or Actrapid), insulin diluent (if needed), insulin pump syringe, an infusion set or catheter, tape (a hypoallergenic type if you are sensitive to regular tape), large-gauge (18- to 20-gauge) disposable needles, and sterile caps for the catheter and syringe.

One of the first steps in preparing a pump involves filling the insulin reservoir. If you use full-strength insulin, use a large-gauge needle to draw it up into the proper syringe. Rid the syringe of any air bubbles and remove the needle. If you dilute the insulin, you can do it either in a syringe or bottle. The syringe technique involves drawing up the prescribed number of insulin units into a syringe and injecting them into the pump syringe. Remove the needle from the insulin pump syringe and pull back the plunger, then inject the insulin into it. Inject slowly and direct the stream to the side of the syringe to avoid introducing air bubbles. Next draw up the prescribed units of insulin diluent into the insulin syringe and again inject it into the pump syringe. Replace the pump syringe needle, rid the solution of any air bubbles, and gently roll the syringe to mix the insulin and diluent.

If you use the bottle technique, start by determining how many units of insulin should be added to 20 milliliters of diluent to produce the proper concentration. Draw the insulin into an insulin syringe and slowly inject it into a 20-milliliter vial of diluent. Draw an equal number of units of air out of the vial to prevent an accumulation of too much pressure in the vial. Roll the solution gently to mix and, using a large-gauge needle, draw the required number of units into the insulin pump syringe. Rid it of any air bubbles. The mixture remaining in the bottle should be stored at room temperature.

After the pump syringe is filled, the next step is to "plant" or attach the pump. Select an infusion site that is convenient (the abdomen, thigh, and hip are favored sites). Attach the syringe and infusion set, flushing the insulin solution through the catheter to rid the system of any air. Cleanse the infusion site with a Betadine swab and allow it to dry. Insert the needle (bevel up) at a forty-five-degree angle into the subcutaneous tissue. Make sure that the needle is horizontal across the body to avoid problems when you bend. After the needle is properly inserted, it should be taped securely in place.

Make sure the pump is set for basal insulin delivery, then mount the syringe on the pump. Recheck all settings; the pump should now be delivering the basal infusion.

To deliver a premeal bolus, start by checking blood sugar thirty to forty-five minutes before the planned meal or snack. Determine how much insulin is needed. (If the blood glucose is more than 150 mg/dl, administer the bolus but delay eating until the glucose level has dropped to 120 mg/dl. If the glucose is lower than 65 mg/dl or there are symptoms of hypoglycemia, administer the bolus and eat immediately. If the symptoms are severe, switch the pump to suspend to temporarily halt the insulin infusion and eat immediately. Restart the insulin infusion when the blood sugar rises to the desired level.) If the glucose is in the normal range, give the bolus and eat thirty minutes later.

OTHER PRECAUTIONS

Check periodically to make sure that there is enough insulin in the syringe. This is particularly important before going to sleep. Check, too, to make sure that there is no insulin seepage. If the needle appears to be slipping out of the infusion site, change it immediately. In any event, the site should be changed every other day, and sites should be rotated to avoid problems of shrinking or hardening of the subcutaneous tissue. If a site is inflamed or painful, contact your doctor. Although the problem of infection can be minimized by following proper procedures, any warning signs should be recognized and treated early. If local allergic reactions occur, try switching tapes. Use a hypoallergenic type that is perforated. Local allergic reactions also may be caused by the insulin or diluent; if so, change either or both as needed.

PUMP PROBLEM SOLVING

A rise or fall in blood sugar may be due to conventional causes— too much or too little exercise, food, or insulin—or they may be caused by a pump malfunction. Most insulin pumps sold today are highly reliable, but as with any machine, mechanical failures can occur. If this happens, contact the nearest manufacturer's representative; many companies will lend a pump while the other is being repaired. However, since most problems encountered with insulin pumps are caused by user error rather than mechanical breakdown, it is a good idea to develop a checklist of potential problem areas and go through it before concluding that the device itself is at fault. Following is a checklist developed by the Diabetes Self-Care Program.

Hyperglycemia

• Disconnected catheter and insulin reservoir. Check that the catheter and insulin reservoir are firmly screwed together.

• Accidental removal of needle from infusion site. Check needle position during each bolus, before going to bed, and upon awakening. The needle should be changed every other day and securely taped.

• Insulin leakage. Check for insulin leakage at the infusion site and also from the catheter. Change the infusion site at prescribed intervals and make sure that the catheter cap is securely connected to the tubing.

• Obstructed insulin flow. Check the catheter for blood clots or precipitation of insulin, which occurs most frequently at the slow basal infusion rates.

• Empty syringe. Check syringe regularly and change at periodic intervals. Have a spare prepared syringe or diluted insulin mixture ready in case of emergencies.

• Incorrect pump setting. Double-check pump settings when administering bolus doses and when changing insulin syringes.

• Power failure. Change batteries as needed and always carry a spare charged battery with you.

• Mechanical failure. Avoid dropping the pump or getting it wet. Return it to the manufacturer for a yearly checkup. Also, select a pump with alarm systems that indicate the nature of the failure (low battery, insulin pump malfunction, etc.).

Hypoglycemia

Wearing an insulin pump does not remove the danger of hypoglycemia from conventional causes, such as delayed or skipped meals (especially if a bolus has been administered), strenuous exercise, or changing hormone levels. Thus, blood glucose should be checked periodically, and food suitable for correcting low blood sugar should always be near at hand, including at the bedside at night. Glucagon also should be available for emergency treatment. Pump-related causes for hypoglycemia include:

- Wrong infusion setting.
- Malfunction of infusion pump controls.

If hypoglycemia occurs, stop the insulin infusion by turning off the pump. You should make sure that there are key people at home and work who know how to turn off the pump and treat hypoglycemia. A tag also should be affixed to the pump giving your doctor's name and phone number, the pump manufacturer's name and phone number, and instructions on how to turn it off in case of emergency.

TEMPORARY DISCONNECTS

After you have stopped taking intermediate- or long-acting insulin and switched over to the pump, any periods during which the pump is disconnected should be managed with Regular or fast-acting insulin. The longer-acting insulins have a carryover effect that makes it difficult to resume pump use. Since there are likely to be many times you will want to remove the device, it is important to know how to handle the situation in advance. Without proper planning, blood sugar will rise about 100 mg/dl per hour when the pump is disconnected. Obviously, this can quickly lead to hyperglycemia unless insulin is administered.

To remove the pump for a short period, say two or three hours, calculate the amount of basal insulin required for the period and administer it as a bolus. (For example, for a 60-kilogram person whose hourly basal infusion is 0.75 units, a bolus of 1.5 units would be required for two hours off the pump.) However, the time limit on such bolus doses is four hours; if the pump is going to be disconnected longer than four hours, Regular insulin should be administered by injection every four hours. Meals consumed during that time should be covered by additional premeal insulin injection. If you plan strenuous exercise, such as a swim or run, while the pump is disconnected, you will require a lesser amount of insulin or more food.

Since the pump should not get wet, it must be removed for bathing, showering, or swimming. A shower or bath can be timed to coincide with changing the infusion site. Alternatively, the pump can be disconnected and the catheter left in place while you shower. However, the catheter also should be removed when you swim.

Many patients hesitate to talk to their doctors about engaging in sexual intercourse while on the pump. Since sex is an important part of a satisfying relationship, both partners should openly discuss this aspect of pump therapy beforehand. With proper planning, the pump should not be a hindrance to a satisfying sexual relationship. Dr. Jovanovic notes that most people prefer to disconnect the pump during sex, at least until both partners are comfortable with the device. If the pump is going to be left off for the entire night, she advises taking the usual before-bed NPH dose, an exception to the rule about not mixing the two insulins. The question of whether a bolus is needed if the pump is going to be reconnected in an hour or two depends on the degree of activity and how long the pump will be off. "If you enjoy sex and are an active participant, it probably is not necessary to bolus," she says. Of course, the question can be resolved by measuring blood sugar before and after, although some people may object to this on the basis that it may spoil some of the romantic aspects of lovemaking. If the pump is left on during sex, it may be advisable to eat a snack first to avoid a possible drop in blood sugar.

THE COST FACTOR

Although a growing number of companies are manufacturing insulin pumps and supplies and prices are coming down, the devices are still expensive. A nonprogrammable pump costs about $1,000 and a programmable one about twice that. In addition, the pumps require batteries, insulin syringes, catheters, and other supplies. Many insurance contracts will cover all or part of these costs; check your policy and make sure that your doctor writes a specific prescription for all the necessary supplies. Even though an insulin pump may cost more than conventional therapy initially, it may produce substantial long-term savings by reducing illness as a result of improved glucose control. Self-Care pump users are advised to have at least a month's supplies—syringes, catheters, batteries, etc.—on hand at all times. Backup batteries and insulin syringes should be kept close at hand, along with the usual blood glucose monitoring supplies. If supplies have to be ordered, do so regularly to ensure that a month's stock is on hand. Some medical supply houses will arrange next-day delivery; check with those in your area to see if this service is available.

SUMMING UP

Portable insulin pumps that can mimic normal pancreatic function more closely than conventional insulin therapy are one of the latest advances in diabetes treatment. Although insulin pumps are not suitable (or necessary) for many people with type 1 diabetes, many others can benefit from their use. These include patients who find it difficult to maintain a consistent, regular life pattern as well as those who have diabetes complications or are at high risk of developing them.

Before switching to pump therapy, you should be well versed in its use. The switchover should be closely supervised, either in a hospital setting or under close outpatient supervision. You should maintain close contact with the physician or other member of the medical team until you are comfortable with the pump and adept at anticipating and preventing possible problems. You also should know how to handle pump emergencies and how to go off the pump if necessary.

9

Managing Pregnancy
Complicated by Diabetes

Perhaps one of the most gratifying achievements in diabetes treatment over the last decade—and one pioneered by researchers at Cornell and Rockefeller universities—has been the development of a regimen that enables a woman with the disease to have a healthy, normal baby. Before the discovery of insulin in 1921, there was no recorded survival of a baby born to a diabetic woman. In the preinsulin era, it was extremely unlikely that a woman with diabetes would become pregnant and, if she did, it was a virtual certainty that the baby would not survive. In many instances, the woman also died.

This grim outlook began to change with the widespread use of insulin, but many problems remained. Only a few years ago, the pregnant woman with diabetes still faced an increased risk of infant mortality—studies conducted in the 1960s and early 1970s showed a mortality rate of up to 21 percent. Among the surviving babies, there was an increased incidence of birth defects: 5 to 18 percent were born with congenital malformations; 20 to 36 percent suffered brain damage; and 2 to 9 percent were born with serious respiratory problems. A large number, 16 to 40 percent, were bigger than normal, weighing in at nine pounds or more at birth. This condition, known as macrosomatia, makes delivery more difficult and raises the risk of death or complications for the baby. What's more, the women themselves risked serious complications, so much so that even before the Supreme Court ruling that legalized abortion, diabetes was a legal justification for terminating a pregnancy because of the danger it posed to the mother.

These unfavorable statistics began to change in the late 1970s with the increased emphasis on tight control of blood sugar. In one of the landmark studies of this period, a group of Cornell and Rockefeller researchers, led by Drs. Jovanovic and Peterson, demonstrated that, if a woman with diabetes maintained normal blood sugar throughout pregnancy, her chances of having a normal baby were the same as those of a nondiabetic woman.

In all, fifty-two diabetic women participated in this study. The opportunity to participate was offered to all diabetic women who were less than twelve weeks pregnant when they first visited The New York Hospital Obstetrical Clinic. Initially, the researchers had planned to divide the women into two groups: half would receive the then-standard care, which involved self-testing of urine for sugar, appropriate insulin and diet, and periodic checkups at the clinic. The other half would be given a more intensive program, developed in an earlier pilot study, which included self-monitoring of blood sugar, a sliding scale of insulin dosages, and meticulous attention to diet and blood sugar control. This plan was discarded after three of the first four babies born to women receiving standard care had severe problems and the fourth was stillborn. "It was decided it would be unethical to continue giving standard care to half the women after it became evident that this protocol, even though it was the accepted treatment, was jeopardizing the well-being of the babies," Dr. Jovanovic explained. As an alternative, all of the diabetic women were switched to the intensive regimen, and their outcome was compared with that of fifty-two nondiabetic women with similar backgrounds, including age, ethnic group, type of delivery (for example, vaginal versus cesarean section), and socioeconomic status.

At the outset, each woman was hospitalized for five to seven days to enable the researchers to normalize blood sugar, to fine-tune the insulin dosage and diet, and to teach the principles of self-care. "Our goal," says Dr. Jovanovic, "was to maintain the mean blood glucose between 80 and 87 mg/dl, with a fasting blood glucose of 55 to 65 mg/dl and the level not exceeding 140 mg/dl an hour after eating, with a goal of 120 mg/dl. In our earlier studies, we had determined that if a woman could maintain a mean blood glucose of about 84 mg/

dl, and not go over the 140 mark, her chances of having a normal baby would be the same as those of a nondiabetic woman."

When the women entered the hospital, their blood sugar levels were considerably higher than the target range: the mean blood glucose before starting the program was 212 mg/dl, and the mean hemoglobin A_{1C} was 10 percent, compared to a normal range of 2 to 5 percent in nondiabetic pregnant women. Those who had complications, such as eye problems or kidney disease, tended to have higher blood sugar than the women with uncomplicated diabetes. But by the time the women were discharged (in most cases, in fewer than seven days), all had blood sugar levels in the target range and all had mastered the principles of self-monitoring and insulin adjustment. "At first, some of our colleagues were skeptical that the women would be able to comply with our protocols," Dr. Jovanovic recalls. "Remember, these were clinic patients; most came from lower socioeconomic groups and half were Hispanic, which might mean some language problems. But they all mastered the program and only two required further hospitalization to resolve questions of blood sugar control."

The outcome astounded critics of the study and more than verified the researchers' hypothesis that maintaining normal blood glucose could produce normal babies despite their mothers' diabetes. All fifty-three babies (one woman had twins) were full-term, and there were no birth defects, respiratory problems, or other abnormalities. In addition, all had perfect Apgar scores five minutes after birth. (This is a standard developed by the late Dr. Virginia Apgar to evaluate the status of the newborn.) In contrast, the fifty-three babies in the nondiabetic comparison group had somewhat lower Apgar scores, five had major congenital malformations, and two had minor defects. "No one had expected our diabetic women to have babies that were actually healthier than those in the comparison group," Dr. Jovanovic recalls. Of course, comparison is difficult, even though the women had many similarities. Dr. Jovanovic explains, "Women in the study received more intensive care, including constant nutritional counseling, than the nondiabetic women. Their postpartum evaluations also were somewhat different."

Even so, the implications of this study for the pregnant woman with diabetes are clear: following the protocols developed for these fifty-two women will greatly enhance the likelihood of having a healthy baby and minimize the hazards to the mother. These protocols, which should be followed only under the direct supervision of a doctor, are described in detail on the following pages. Several other medical centers also have developed protocols for managing diabetes during pregnancy; while there may be some slight differences in details, all embrace the principle verified in the Cornell-Rockefeller program: *a normal blood sugar is the key to a good outcome in the pregnancy of diabetic women.*

PLANNING BEFORE PREGNANCY

Despite the tremendous advances in managing the pregnancy of diabetic women and the improved outlook for both mother and baby, couples should realize that it is still a very demanding endeavor. "A woman has to be very motivated and conscientious," Dr. Jovanovic stresses. "Fortunately, our most motivated and determined patients are diabetic women who want to be mothers."

Ideally, the program of normalizing blood sugar should be mastered before pregnancy begins. This means practicing blood glucose self-monitoring and knowing how to match insulin, food, and exercise to control blood sugar. "We would like to see our mothers maintain normal blood sugar for at least three months before conception takes place," Dr. Jovanovic says. "The healthier a woman is before getting pregnant, the better her outlook." The Diabetes Self-Care Program has a special prepregnancy component designed to help women achieve this goal.

Before attempting a pregnancy, the diabetic woman should consult with her doctor, who should carefully evaluate her for complications that might be exacerbated by pregnancy. Several classifications to help doctors identify the problem areas in diabetic pregnancies have been developed (see Tables 1 to 3). Since pregnancy sometimes causes a worsening of certain complications, such as retinopathy, kidney disease, high blood pressure, and coronary artery disease, it is important to be aware of any such problems before attempting a pregnancy. If there are serious complications, the woman may be advised to delay pregnancy until they can be brought under control; there also may be situations in which pregnancy would pose too great a risk to the mother's health.

TABLE 1

WHITE CLASSIFICATION
OF PREGNANCIES OF DIABETIC WOMEN

Category	Definition
A	Abnormal glucose tolerance test, but no symptoms. Normal blood glucose can be maintained by diet without insulin therapy
B	Onset of diabetes after age 20, with a duration of less than 10 years
C	Onset of diabetes at relatively young age (10 to 19) or of relatively long duration (10 to 19 years)
D	Onset at a very early age (less than 10 years) or very long duration (20 or more years) or evidence of retinopathy
F	Kidney disease
R	Proliferative retinopathy
RF	Both renal disease and proliferative retinopathy
G	Multiple reproductive failures, such as habitual miscarriages and/or stillbirths
H	Arteriosclerotic heart disease
T	Pregnancy after kidney transplant

Adapted from Lois Jovanovic and Charles M. Peterson, "Modern Monitoring and Management of the Diabetic Pregnant Patient," in *Modern Management of High-Risk Pregnancy*, edited by Niels H. Lauersen. New York: Plenum, 1983.

TABLE 2

DEFINITIONS OF DIABETES CONTROL

Criteria for good diabetes control:
    Fasting blood glucose of 55 to 65 mg/dl
    Mean 24-hour blood glucose of 80 to 87 mg/dl
    Blood glucose of 120 mg/dl or lower 1 hour after meal
    Normal glycohemoglobin: HbA_{1C} up to 5%

Less than optimal diabetes control:
    Pregnancies in which the glucose control was not documented
    Pregnancies in which glucose control was outside the normal range
    Good control not established by or maintained after 2 weeks in gestational diabetes or diabetic women with abnormal glycosylated hemoglobin at time of conception

Adapted from Lois Jovanovic and Charles M. Peterson, "Modern Monitoring and Management of the Diabetic Pregnant Patient," in *Modern Management of High-Risk Pregnancy*, edited by Niels H. Lauersen. New York: Plenum, 1983.

TABLE 3

PYKE CLASSIFICATION
OF DIABETES IN PREGNANCY

Type	Definition
Gestational	Diabetes that starts during pregnancy and disappears after delivery
Pregestational	Diabetes that begins before conception and continues after pregnancy
Complicated pregestational	Diabetes complicated by vascular diseases, such as nephropathy, retinopathy, or peripheral vascular disease

Adapted from Lois Jovanovic and Charles M. Peterson, "Modern Monitoring and Management of the Diabetic Pregnant Patient," in *Modern Management of High-Risk Pregnancy*, edited by Niels Lauersen. New York: Plenum, 1983.

Even in the absence of any complications, pregnancy has a profound effect on diabetes and insulin uptake. For example, the placenta produces hormones and enzymes that either are antagonistic to insulin or increase its degradation. In addition, carbohydrate metabolism changes during pregnancy, probably because of the elevated levels of estrogen and progesterone; therefore, both fasting and average blood glucose levels should be lower during pregnancy than at other times. Blood glucose passes freely to the developing fetus but the mother's insulin does not. If the fetal blood glucose is too high, the baby's pancreas will try to compensate by producing insulin. Since insulin is also a growth hormone, it is one of the factors that produces oversize babies. Also, the extra insulin and high blood glucose tend to lower the baby's potassium level, which leads to flaccid muscles and can cause fatal arrhythmias. In short, normal glucose levels are never more important than during pregnancy, yet they may be harder to achieve.

Since a diabetic pregnancy is time-consuming for both the woman and her physician, it is important to make sure that the doctor is experienced in this area and willing to expend the extra effort. Ideally, the medical care should be a team effort, involving an obstetrician to manage the pregnancy; an internist, endocrinologist, or diabetologist to manage the diabetes; a dietitian for nutritional counseling; and perhaps a diabetes educator or nurse experienced in this area to help coordinate the efforts and provide special services as needed. "It is vital that the woman be able to reach her doctor or someone who is standing in for the doctor at all times," Dr. Jovanovic states. In fact, Dr. Jovanovic gives her patients regular telephone appointments so she can keep extra-close watch over them between office visits, and she encourages them to call her "even in the middle of the night or on weekends" at the first hint of anything amiss.

Even though a whole team of doctors and other health professionals may be involved, Dr. Jovanovic emphasizes that "the patient has to be in command." As in all facets of effective self-care, this involves careful self-monitoring of blood glucose and knowing how to anticipate and solve problems before they occur.

In the initial Cornell-Rockefeller pregnancy studies, the women spent a week in the hospital undergoing a thorough medical evaluation and learning all aspects of self-care. This is still recommended, but if hospitalization is not practical or feasible, the evaluation can be made and the protocols taught on an outpatient basis.

The medical evaluation includes a complete physical examination, with particular attention paid to the cardiovascular system, kidneys, eyes, and neurological status. A number of tests will be performed, including routine blood and urine studies. (These are repeated at all subsequent visits.) An accurate dating of pregnancy also is important. Self-Care patients in the prepregnancy program are taught to chart their basal temperatures to identify the time of ovulation, an important factor since many diabetic women have irregular menstrual cycles.

CALCULATING INSULIN DOSAGE

After the medical evaluation, the next steps are to establish an optimum insulin regimen and to match this with a diet. The total insulin dosage is based on body weight and stage of pregnancy. This varies from woman to woman, but the general formula followed by the Self-Care Program calls for 0.7 units per kilogram of body weight per twenty-four hours for the first twelve weeks; 0.8 units per kilogram for weeks twelve to twenty-four; 0.9 units for weeks twenty-four to thirty-six; and 1.0 unit per kilogram from the thirty-sixth week until delivery. This is divided into three doses, along the lines described in Chapter 5. The regimen followed in the Cornell-Rockefeller pregnancy study called for a combination of NPH and Regular insulins, although other short- and intermediate-acting insulins, such as Semilente or Lente, may be prescribed. Self-Care obstetrical patients are taught to adjust their insulin according to the rule of eighteens. The total insulin dosage is divided into eighteenths and administered as follows:

Type of Insulin	7:30 A.M.	4:30 P.M.	10 P.M.
NPH	8/18		3/18
Regular	4/18	3/18	
Total	2/3	1/6	1/6

An example of how this works is: Assume the woman weighs 121 pounds or 55 kilograms. Her total daily insulin requirement for the first twelve weeks of pregnancy would be 55 × 0.7 or 38.5 units. Using the rule of eighteens, the dosage would be:

Type of Insulin	7:30 A.M.	4:30 P.M.	10 P.M.
NPH	18		6
Regular	9	6	

By the second trimester, let's assume that the woman has gained 1 kilogram and her insulin need has increased to 0.8 units per kilogram. Her basic dosage would then become:

Type of Insulin	7:30 A.M.	4:30 P.M.	10 P.M.
NPH	20		7
Regular	10	7	

As pregnancy progresses, and the woman enters the third trimester, let's assume her weight has increased to 60 kilograms and she now requires 0.9 units of insulin per kilogram. The basic dosage would increase to:

Type of Insulin	7:30 A.M.	4:30 P.M.	10 P.M.
NPH	24		9
Regular	12	9	

By the thirty-seventh week of pregnancy, she weighs 64 kilograms and her insulin requirement has increased to 1.0 unit per kilogram. The basic dosage would be adjusted to:

Type of Insulin	7:30 A.M.	4:30 P.M.	10 P.M.
NPH	28		11
Regular	14	11	

Once the basic dosage is established, the Regular dosage is adjusted according to the following sliding scale, depending on specific blood glucose measurements.

Regular Insulin Adjustment According to Rule of Eighteens

If 7:30 A.M. blood sugar is:	If 4:30 P.M. blood sugar is:
Under 60 mg/dl, give 3/18 of total calculated dose	under 60 mg/dl, give 2/18 of total calculated dose
60–100 mg/dl, give 4/18	60–100 mg/dl, give 3/18
100–140 mg/dl,* give 5/18	100–140 mg/dl,* give 4/18
Over 140 mg/dl,* give 6/18	Over 140 mg/dl,* give 5/18

* Note: this applies to readings on a glucose meter. If visual strips are used, lower value to 120 mg/dl.

In practice, the sliding scale for the 55-kilogram woman described earlier might be as follows:

The 7:30 A.M. fasting blood glucose is 120; the morning Regular is increased to 5/18, or 11 units. But if the blood glucose is 55, the morning Regular is decreased to 3/18, or 6 units. Similar adjustments would be made in the before-dinner Regular dose, in line with the 4:30 P.M. glucose. (Other protocols for adjusting insulin and diet are given in Table 4.)

CALCULATING THE DIET

Dietary needs, like those for insulin, change as pregnancy progresses. If the woman's weight is in the normal range (80 to 120 percent of ideal weight for age and body type), the daily calorie re-

TABLE 4

PROTOCOL FOR ADJUSTING INSULIN AND DIET

Blood Sugar		Regular Insulin		NPH Insulin		Diet Adjustment
Time	Level	Time	Dose	Time	Dose	
7:30 A.M.	<60	7:30 A.M.	−2 U*	10 P.M.	−2 U	
	60–100	(same day)	no change	(same day)	no change	
Fasting	100–140†		+2 U		+2 U	
	>140†		+4 U		+4 U	
10 A.M.	>140†	7:30 A.M. next day	+2 U			Skip 10:30 A.M. snack today
Noon	<60					Add 100 calories to 10:30 A.M. snack next day
1 P.M.	>140†					Skip 3 P.M. snack today

Time	Blood glucose	4:30 P.M. same day	7:30 A.M. next day	4:30 P.M. next day	
4 P.M.	<60	−2 U	−2 U		
	60–100	no change	no change		
	100–140†	+2 U	+2 U		
	>140†	+4 U	+4 U		
6 P.M.	>140†			+2 U	Skip 8 P.M. snack today
8 P.M.	<60			−2 U	
	60–140†			no change	
	>140†			+2 U	
10 P.M.	>100				Skip 11 P.M. snack today

* Adjustments are plus or minus regular calculated dose.

† When using visually read strips, use 120 mg/dl value.

Adapted from "Protocols for Managing Diabetes in Pregnancy, A Guide for Physicians and Allied Healthcare Professionals," prepared by Drs. Lois Jovanovic, Carol B. Braun, Maurice L. Druzin, and Charles M. Peterson.

quirements are calculated at 25 calories per kilogram prior to pregnancy and early in the first trimester and 30 calories per kilogram thereafter. (For women who are more than 20 percent above their ideal weight, the calorie allowance may be somewhat lower; say, 24 calories per kilogram. However, caution must be used to make sure that the woman does not begin breaking down stored body fat, a situation that may produce ketone bodies in the blood and urine.) Using this formula, the woman who begins pregnancy at a normal weight of 55 kilograms will require 1,375 calories a day for the first twelve weeks and, as weight is gained thereafter, 30 calories per kilogram of present body weight until delivery. This should produce a total weight gain of 22 to 26 pounds, an ideal increase for a pregnant woman. The calorie allotment and recommended weight gain are about the same as for nondiabetic women; however, the diabetic woman must be much more precise in the way she distributes calories among the three classes of nutrients and also in the timing of meals. The nutrient distribution is the same as that recommended for all patients with type 1 diabetes: 40 percent of the total calories should come from carbohydrates, 20 percent from protein, and 40 percent from fat. (See Chapter 6 for details of how to calculate the proper amounts of food.)

The distribution of calories into meals is somewhat different: for pregnant patients, Dr. Jovanovic again advocates that calories be distributed according to the rule of eighteens, which is summarized as follows:

INITIAL DISTRIBUTION OF CALORIES

Time	Meal	Fraction of Day's Calories
8 A.M.	Breakfast	2/18
10:30 A.M.	Snack	1/18
Noon	Lunch	5/18
3 P.M.	Snack	2/18
5 P.M.	Dinner	5/18
8 P.M.	Snack	2/18
11 P.M.	Snack	1/18

While this may seem like a lot of calculating, it actually is quite simple, especially with the help of a calculator and calorie charts. Maintaining a careful daily diary is especially important during pregnancy: a sample record sheet is included in this chapter.

GLUCOSE SELF-MONITORING

Since an accurate blood glucose profile is essential in making the necessary insulin and food adjustments, at least six to eight measurements should be taken each day throughout the pregnancy. These are:

- 7:30 A.M., or upon arising, which is the fasting blood glucose
- 9:30 A.M., or one hour after breakfast
- 1 P.M., or an hour after lunch
- 4:30 P.M., or an hour before dinner
- 6:30 P.M., or an hour after dinner
- 10 P.M., or at bedtime

Other measurements that may be required, particularly in the beginning, include:

- 3 A.M. Blood sugar tends to be its lowest at about this time. A glucose check will determine whether additional food should be taken before going to bed and whether the bedtime insulin dosage should be adjusted.
- 11 A.M. This will tell whether the midmorning snack is adequate to cover the peaking of the morning Regular insulin.
- 8 P.M. This will indicate whether calories should be shifted from dinner to an evening snack to cover the peaking of the predinner Regular insulin.

Of course, a glucose measurement should be taken if symptoms of low or high blood sugar occur. Measurements before and after exercise also may be important.

URINE TESTING

In addition to measuring blood glucose, patients also are instructed to test their urine for acetone (or ketones) at least every morning and perhaps more often. Diabetic pregnant women should be particularly careful not to skip meals or skimp on their daily food intake. Nonpregnant patients can get away with this by adjusting their insulin and exercise, but during pregnancy, one of the goals is to avoid producing ketones—the acid substances that are a by-product of the breakdown of fatty tissue that occurs during a state of semistarvation. Blood glucose may be normal even though the woman is approaching a state of ketoacidosis. Ketones pass into the fetal circulation, and while it is controversial whether they cause any lasting damage to the baby, it is advisable to avoid exposing the fetus to them. Even obese women should not try to lose weight during pregnancy. The frequent small meals are intended to provide a steady source of glucose without the need to break down stored body fat and exposing the baby to potentially harmful ketones. "Some women may need to eat even more often than the usual three-meal, four-snack schedule," Dr. Jovanovic notes. "A high acetone level in the morning may indicate the woman should have a snack in the middle of the night—eight hours without food may be too long."

CHECKING FETAL DEVELOPMENT

While following the Cornell-Rockefeller protocol maximizes the chances of having a healthy baby, frequent checkups to make sure all is going well are very important. This may mean seeing the doctor or visiting the obstetrical clinic weekly. At each visit, the woman's daily diary of blood glucose levels, urine acetone tests, insulin dosages, and other pertinent details should be reviewed and further adjustments made, if indicated. To double-check blood sugar control, glycohemoglobin should be measured at least once a month. Several sonograms may be made during the course of pregnancy: one in the first trimester and again between eighteen and twenty-four weeks. Urine will be checked for acetone, protein, and other signs of kidney problems. Periodic urine cultures for urinary tract infections also should be made. Special attention should be paid to blood pressure and other signs of potential problems, such as accumulation of body fluids. The woman also should see her opthalmologist periodically throughout her pregnancy.

The pregnant woman also should know when to expect certain indications of normal fetal development. Quickening, the early fluttering sensations of fetal movement, should occur between the eighteenth and twentieth weeks of a first pregnancy, and between the sixteenth and eighteenth weeks in subsequent ones. The doctor should begin to hear the fetal heartbeat with a fetoscope at about eighteen weeks. (A Doppler device can detect the fetal heartbeat at eleven weeks' gestation.)

As pregnancy nears term, fetal movements are an important index of the baby's health: the more activity the better. After thirty-two weeks, the woman should make a daily check of fetal movements. This can be done in one of two ways. At a specific time each day, the woman should lie on her side, with her chest and head propped up at a forty-five-degree angle. All movements—kicks, rolls, hiccups, etc.—should be counted. If there are fewer than four in an hour, the woman should call her doctor immediately. From the thirty-sixth week on, the fetal movements should be checked twice a day; after the thirty-eighth week, three times a day. Three half-hour periods can be set aside (one each in the morning, midday, and evening) for the counting. A running total should be kept for each day. If there are fewer than ten movements, a doctor should be called.

In Case of Hypoglycemia

Any blood sugar level outside the normal range should be avoided during pregnancy; just as too much blood glucose is harmful, so is too little. Women who follow a program of tight control are not as likely to develop hypoglycemia as are those under less than optimal control, but the possibility cannot be overlooked. Since hypoglycemia can sometimes progress rapidly to coma, pregnant women should be particularly attuned to the warning signs (see page 66–67). If a woman suspects her blood sugar is falling too low, she should immediately check it. If it is less than 70 mg/dl with a glucose meter or between 40 and 80 with visual strips, she should drink an 8-ounce glass of whole milk, which provides about 12 grams of carbohydrates plus protein for a slower source of glucose. The milk should increase blood glucose by about 30 mg/dl in fifteen minutes. To make sure, blood sugar should be measured again fifteen minutes after drinking the milk. If the glucose is still below 70 mg/dl, a second glass of milk should be consumed, with another check of blood sugar in fifteen minutes. If the sugar is still below 70 mg/dl, a slice of bread and a third glass of milk should be consumed.

If the blood sugar cannot be elevated by eating—for example, many women experience nausea and vomiting in the first few months of pregnancy—an injection of glucagon should be used. A subcutaneous injection of 0.15 mg (or 15 "units" in an insulin syringe) of glucagon should raise blood sugar 30 to 40 mg/dl. Glucagon also can be administered if hypoglycemia has progressed to the point where the woman is unable to measure her blood sugar or think clearly. A fresh syringe of glucagon always should be on hand and husbands or other members of the household should know how to use it in case of emergency.

USE OF AN INSULIN PUMP DURING PREGNANCY

The development of increasingly reliable insulin pumps provides the pregnant woman and her medical team with an alternative method of insulin therapy. Since an insulin pump can be programmed to continuously administer small amounts of insulin to cover basal needs and larger basal infusions to cover meals, it would seem logical that this would make it easier to achieve the kind of tight control of blood sugar that is so important during pregnancy. While studies have shown that a normal blood sugar profile can be achieved more readily with an insulin pump than through periodic injections, there are certain hazards to using an insulin pump during pregnancy. Hypoglycemia, especially during the early morning hours when the body is likely to be its most insulin-resistant, is more likely to occur with an insulin pump because there is no reserve of slow- or intermediate-acting insulin in the body. Of course, the more advanced types of insulin pumps can be programmed to deliver extra insulin at about 3 A.M.; if an insulin pump is used during pregnancy, it should be the type that can be programmed to increase or decrease basal infusions as needed.

Pump failure is another potentially serious problem. If an insulin pump accidentally becomes disconnected while the woman is asleep, the results can be disastrous for both the mother and baby. Therefore, the woman should plan to wake up during the night to check that the pump is connected and functioning properly. The pump also should be the type with automatic alarms that signal an accidental disconnect or other failure.

While stressing these potential hazards, Dr. Jovanovic notes that there are some pregnant women for whom an insulin pump may be an acceptable alternative to conventional therapy. "If a woman is on the pump before becoming pregnant and is comfortable and skilled in its use, then there probably is no reason to change during pregnancy," she explains. An insulin pump also may be time-saving and help some women achieve better control of their diabetes. "The key is a thorough understanding of what is involved in using an insulin pump," Dr. Jovanovic emphasizes. "It does not remove the need for careful self-monitoring of blood sugar, nor does it guarantee better glucose control. But if it is well understood, it can be a highly useful tool for the pregnant woman."

GESTATIONAL DIABETES

Gestational diabetes occurs during pregnancy and disappears almost immediately after delivery. It is estimated that 2 to 6 percent of all pregnant women may have gestational diabetes, and in many it is not identified in time to prevent its complications. Routine urine and blood glucose tests often are not enough to identify women with gestational diabetes, especially if they were tested in a fasting state. Dr. Jovanovic explains, "Most pregnant women know they are going to be put on the scale when they see their obstetricians and if they have gained too much weight, they will expect to be scolded. So the natural reaction is to starve for a day or so before seeing the doctor." The resulting blood glucose test may be in the normal range, but higher than normal for a fasting state. If the doctor is unaware that it is, indeed, a fasting level, the results are easily misinterpreted.

Since gestational diabetes is now known to be much more common than once thought, a number of experts, including the Cornell-Rockefeller researchers, advocate that all pregnant women be screened for it, usually in the twenty-sixth week of pregnancy. The screening test involves giving the woman a drink containing 50 grams of glucose and then measuring the blood sugar an hour later. If the plasma glucose is more than 150 mg/dl, a three-hour glucose tolerance test with 100 grams of oral glucose is administered. If the results of this test are positive, treatment to normalize blood glucose should begin immediately. In some cases, diet alone may be enough to bring the blood sugar into the normal range; if not, the woman should undergo the same treatment as the pregnant woman with type 1 diabetes. In either event, these women should be taught glucose self-monitoring and keep a careful diary.

A number of factors that increase the risk of gestational diabetes have been identified.

- A family history of diabetes (including distant relatives)
- A history of sugar in the urine
- A history of glucose intolerance
- Obesity (more than 20 percent above ideal body weight)
- Patient's own birthweight of more than 9 pounds
- A poor obstetrical history, including habitual miscarriages, still-births, congenital defects, previous large babies, toxemia, polyhydramnios (excessive amniotic fluid) or recurrent urinary tract infections during pregnancy.

Women who fall into any of these high-risk categories probably should be screened for gestational diabetes more often; for example, in the twelfth, eighteenth, and thirty-second weeks of pregnancy.

Although gestational diabetes disappears after delivery, these women should be followed carefully during any future pregnancy. Also, they are at higher risk of developing diabetes later and therefore should be alert to any symptoms of the disease.

As Delivery Nears

Because of the high incidence of stillbirths or third-trimester fetal death, doctors in the past have been reluctant to let a diabetic woman's pregnancy proceed to full term. The woman would be admitted to the hospital for early delivery, either by cesarean section or induced labor, during the thirty-fifth to thirty-eighth weeks of pregnancy. However, this strategy often resulted in delivering premature babies whose lungs were not fully developed (hyaline membrane disease).

Today, the preferred approach is to keep very close watch over the woman throughout the third trimester, particularly from the thirty-fourth week of pregnancy onward. If the woman has maintained normal blood glucose throughout her pregnancy, the chances are good that she will proceed to full term and a normal delivery. Even though this is the expected outcome, Self-Care physicians urge erring on the side of caution and not taking any unnecessary chances. In addition to having the mother check fetal movement daily, doctors also may want to assess the fetal heart rate. This involves documenting whether the baby's heart rate increases after fetal movement; if it does, studies have found that the chance of stillbirth within the next seven days is less than 1 percent. Drs. Jovanovic and Peterson advocate that this nonstress test of the fetal heart rate be performed "any time the mother reports a sudden decrease in fetal movements, a drop in her usual insulin requirement, or any change in her clinical condition."

Because this test may give a false diagnosis of fetal distress 25 to

40 percent of the time, two abnormal tests should be recorded before proceeding to delivery of a mature fetus. Maturity can be determined by tests of the amniotic fluid, which should be done after thirty-six to thirty-seven weeks of pregnancy. If these tests indicate the lungs are not fully developed, another study, a contraction stress test, is advised in addition to the heart rate assessments. The contraction test involves inducing uterine contractions to determine whether a problem of insufficiency in the uterus or placenta is causing the abnormal fetal heart response. If this test is also positive, and fetal death appears imminent, the best decision might be to deliver the baby, even though it may be necessary to treat respiratory difficulties and other problems of immaturity.

As soon as tests show the fetal lungs are mature enough to function on their own, most doctors prefer to deliver the baby as soon as possible. This usually means inducing labor, although a cesarean section may be preferred under some circumstances. In any event, maintaining normal blood glucose throughout labor and delivery remains a top priority. "It would be tragic to work so hard to stay on an even keel throughout pregnancy and then have something happen at the end through loss of control," Dr. Jovanovic observes. She tells her patients to be prepared to continue their own self-care even while in the hospital to give birth. Just before birth, insulin requirements are usually relatively high, but when active labor is established (defined as three contractions of one minute each every ten minutes), insulin requirements fall to zero while glucose needs increase to 2.55 milligrams per kilogram per minute. This is provided by glucose infusion. Blood glucose should be checked regularly throughout labor to make sure that it stays in the 80- to 100-mg/dl range.

If an elective cesarean section is to be performed, the same goal of maintaining normal blood glucose prevails. The usual dose of NPH is taken the night before the operation and repeated the next morning (and every eight hours thereafter if surgery is delayed). Blood sugar should be monitored during the surgery, and any adjustments in insulin or glucose made to maintain the blood sugar between 80 and 100 mg/dl.

AFTER DELIVERY

Immediately after delivery, insulin requirements usually drop greatly and remain low for up to ninety-six hours. Women with gestational diabetes may not need any further insulin injections, although a three-hour glucose tolerance test is advisable six weeks after delivery or when she is no longer breast-feeding.

Mothers who had diabetes before pregnancy will have to start treatment again, usually within a few days of delivery. Insulin should be resumed when the blood glucose rises to 160 mg/dl or more an hour after eating or when the fasting level is greater than 110 mg/dl. The daily dosage should return to 0.6 units of insulin per kilogram of postpartum weight.

The calorie requirements also return to the prepregnancy ratio of 25 calories per kilogram per day, unless the woman elects to breast-feed. In that case, the daily calorie requirements are increased to 27 per kilogram per day. The insulin requirement may drop to less than 0.6 units per day. Part of the decreased insulin requirement is noted overnight when the nursing baby siphons glucose from the mother at a time when she may not be eating.

SPECIAL PRECAUTIONS FOR THE BABY

All pregnancies of diabetic women are considered high-risk; consequently, the babies usually are treated as high-risk infants until it is proved otherwise. A pediatrician experienced in handling high-risk babies should be on hand for the delivery. If normal blood sugar has been maintained throughout the pregnancy and the baby is carried to full term and delivered without signs of respiratory distress or other problems, the baby can be treated like any other normal newborn. This was the situation with all of the babies born to the fifty-two women in the Cornell-Rockefeller study described earlier and, according to Dr. Jovanovic, "We can now assume a more relaxed attitude toward babies born to women who had documented normal blood sugar while pregnant."

The situation is somewhat different if blood sugar control has been less than optimal, however. In this situation, it is a good idea to keep the baby in an intensive-care unit for at least twenty-four hours so he or she can be observed for any problems. The baby's blood glucose should be checked every six hours during this period; he or she also should be watched for signs of respiratory distress or metabolic disturbances. If no problems develop during the first twenty-four hours, the baby can then be placed in a regular nursery.

SUMMING UP

The major factor determining whether a woman with diabetes will have a normal baby is meticulous control of blood sugar throughout pregnancy, labor, and delivery. A number of studies, including a major one involving Diabetes Self-Care Program physicians, have demonstrated that women who have normal blood sugar throughout pregnancy do not have any increased risk of fetal death or congenital defects. Maintaining this kind of control requires frequent self-testing of blood sugar and knowing how to adjust insulin and diet to keep it in the desired range. Most women can master the necessary techniques, but considerable motivation and time are required. However, as Dr. Jovanovic notes, "I've never had a patient who didn't think the reward of having a healthy baby was not worth the effort."

SAMPLE RECORD SHEET FOR USE DURING PREGNANCY

DATE	BLOOD GLUCOSE LEVELS									URINE ACETONE (RESULT & TIME)		INSULIN DOSAGE			NOTES: include insulin reactions; diet changes; feelings of hunger and fatigue; times of hypo- and hyperglycemic episodes; and corrective measures taken.
	BRKFST		LUNCH		DINNER		BED-TIME	OTHER (TIME)		AM	PM	TIME	NPH	Reg	
	B	A	B	A	B	A									

Adapted from *Your Guide to a Healthy Happy Pregnancy*, by Lois Jovanovic, M.D. Copyright Bio-Dynamics. Reprinted with permission of Boehringer Mannheim.

II

Complications of Diabetes

Since diabetes is a metabolic disorder affecting the entire body, it is understandable that it can lead to many different long-term complications involving a number of organs. In earlier chapters, we have discussed the more immediate problems involving blood glucose levels that are either too high or too low. Most people with diabetes can avoid these primary problems by following a good program of blood glucose control. Unfortunately, tight blood glucose control may not always prevent some of the long-term, secondary complications, although recent research indicates that some may be reversed, minimized, or delayed by maintaining normal blood sugar. In this section, we will review the major long-term complications of diabetes and offer guidance from the Diabetes Self-Care Program on how they can be treated or perhaps avoided.

Not all people with diabetes develop these secondary disorders; many have lived with the disease for decades without major complications. But some people have complications that seem to be unrelated to the degree of control or even duration of the disease. While this unfortunate course may be the exception, especially in well-controlled diabetes, doctors are unable to predict who is likely to develop certain complications and who will escape them. Therefore, you should see your doctor regularly and also be alert to warning signs that may herald complications. The longer a secondary complication goes untreated, the more likely it is to become irreversible; thus early diagnosis and treatment are especially important.

A moderate, healthy lifestyle, while important for everyone, is even more so for the person with diabetes. For example, excessive stress is believed to increase the risk of illness for the population as a whole, but the person with diabetes subjected to stress encounters an almost immediate rise in blood glucose. Health authorities agree that cigarette smoking is the leading preventable cause of illness and premature death in this country, accounting for about 120,000 cancer deaths a year and more than 225,000 deaths from cardiovascular disease. Since those with diabetes already have a high risk of heart attacks and stroke, smoking simply compounds the risk. Diet is also a major factor in cardiovascular disease, contributing to an increased risk from high cholesterol, obesity, and perhaps high blood pressure. Since people with diabetes tend to have elevated cholesterol and triglycerides, and type 2 diabetic patients are often overweight, it again makes sense to avoid compounding risks as much as possible by paying close attention to diet and taking other preventive measures, such as exercise conditioning.

As emphasized throughout this book, the prudent lifestyle advocated by the Diabetes Self-Care Program is not one of denial and longing for forbidden pleasures. It is one of moderation that allows you the flexibility needed to live as normal and as rewarding a life as possible. Dr. Peterson repeatedly tells patients that they can eat and do almost anything as long as it is done in moderation and with proper planning. Self-Care patients repeatedly demonstrate that they can have interesting and dynamic careers, rear families, travel, eat in fine restaurants, engage in all kinds of sports, and live remarkably normal lives, even if complications do occur. John, a physician from Pittsburgh who has had diabetes since his teens, says most people, including many with diabetes, have difficulty understanding this. "Even now, whenever I go home, my mother wants to know what I can eat and keeps urging me to rest," he says. "She simply doesn't understand that I can eat everything the rest of the family eats, and that sitting around taking it easy is actually bad for my health. I think it's safe to say that my lifestyle is healthier than that of 90 percent of the general population, despite the fact I have an incurable disease." John is convinced that his healthy lifestyle is helping prevent many of the complications of diabetes, even though there is no scientific evidence that this is necessarily so. But "no matter what," he adds, "I know I feel better because I am in good physical condition. This alone justifies the effort."

As emphasized in the following chapters, a growing number of researchers and other diabetes experts are now convinced that many of the complications of diabetes can be forestalled or minimized by a common-sense approach and by diligent self-care. This involves not only careful monitoring and control of blood sugar but also attention to such things as regular eye examinations, foot care, and good personal hygiene to avoid infection. No one can promise that you still will not encounter problems, but the risk is lower, and a healthy attitude and feeling of being in control can make coping with these problems easier.

10

Psychological Aspects of Diabetes

Any chronic disease raises havoc with the emotional well-being of both the patient and people close to him or her. This is particularly true of diabetes, a disease that requires almost constant attention and that has a profound effect on virtually every aspect of day-to-day life. Feelings of anger, depression, anxiety, hopelessness, frustration, and worthlessness are common, and, in the view of some doctors, almost to be expected. Many patients have recurring thoughts of suicide; others become obsessed with their symptoms, and still others are overcome by feelings of guilt or paranoia. "Why me?" is a frequent and understandable response.

Yet many people with severe diabetes lead productive, rewarding lives, complete with close personal relationships, fulfilling careers, and interesting hobbies. Says Dr. Jovanovic, "I tell patients we must not become preoccupied with thinking of ourselves as 'diabetics.' Instead, we are physicians, musicians, parents, joggers—what have you—who also happen to have diabetes."

It would be a mistake, however, to imply that the emotional effects of diabetes are largely a matter of attitude and positive thinking. While these may be important, the disease itself, particularly the fluctuating levels of blood sugar, can produce psychological effects. Mood changes, feelings of anxiety, irritability, and other psychological changes accompany variations in blood sugar. Patients with poorly controlled blood sugar often describe jarring mood swings, from feelings of euphoria to depression as blood sugar rises and falls. "They also feel they have no control and a lack of control can be depressing to anyone, with or without diabetes," Dr. Peterson explains. "Very often they lack the skills or training to control their diabetes; even though they work very hard to follow instructions, they still have poor control and don't know how to correct this. Understandably, this leads to feelings of helplessness and frustration."

All this can become something of a vicious cycle. Out-of-control diabetes can produce negative psychological responses; in turn, these reactions can affect blood sugar and further interfere with control. Dr. Jovanovic illustrates this point by recalling the experience of a patient in her pregnancy study. "She was in the hospital awaiting the birth of her baby. She also had a pregnant poodle at home that she was very concerned about. When it came time for the poodle to deliver, she asked to go home for the happy event. When she left the hospital, her blood sugar was absolutely normal and she was in great shape. She returned a couple of hours later with a blood sugar of more than 300 mg/dl and obviously very upset. All the puppies had been stillborn, which shows what an emotional upset can do to blood sugar."

A number of researchers have documented the effects of stress on blood sugar. There is also increasing medical and scientific awareness of the effects of stress on overall health. Studies have linked excessive stress or, perhaps more correctly, inability to effectively cope with stress, with a variety of disorders, including an increased risk of heart attacks, high blood pressure, and a number of autoimmune diseases.

An individual's response to stress produces a number of measurable physical changes. One of the most obvious reactions to stress is the classic fight or flight response, which is the body's way of protecting itself from danger. There is a sudden increase in adrenaline or epinephrine, a hormone that increases heart rate, blood pressure, and blood sugar, among other bodily changes. The adrenal glands also release extra cortisone, which increases blood sugar by inhibiting the action of insulin. These changes are intended to give a person the sudden extra energy to overcome a potential danger, and usually pass once the perceived danger or stress is resolved. But some people respond to even minor annoyances as if they were major dangers or stresses. A certain amount of stress is unavoidable; indeed, some people actually seem to thrive on stress; they perform best when pressed by deadlines and demands of work or family. Others seem to lose control when faced with even minor stresses.

Personality type seems to have a good deal to do with our ability to cope with stress; a number of studies have found that people with type A personality—people who tend to be time-driven, ambitious, aggressive, compulsive, always on the go—have a greater risk of heart attacks and certain other illnesses than the calmer, less hurried type B's. Studies also have found that people subjected to a good deal of stress have an increased risk of developing type 2 diabetes. There is a specific type of diabetes that appears to be directly related to excessive stress and disappears once the stress is removed. Since stress has such definite, measurable effects on the body, including hormone levels directly related to blood sugar, it is understandable that diabetic patients who are subjected to considerable stress or who have difficulty in coping with it also have difficulty controlling blood sugar. Simply having a chronic disease like diabetes that requires constant attention to even the most routine aspects of daily life in itself produces extra stress. But it is important that diabetic patients recognize the extra hazards that stress poses for them and learn effective means of stress management. Exercise, meditation, biofeedback training, and behavior modification are among the many approaches to stress management now available.

GOOD CONTROL AND WELL-BEING

Studies by Rockefeller and Cornell physicians have documented that good control of diabetes results in enhanced mental health, even though achieving this kind of control involves careful self-monitoring of blood sugar. When self-testing of blood glucose was first introduced, many physicians expressed reservations about the psychological effect this might have on patients. Some doctors still feel that frequent self-testing may lead to undue preoccupation with symptoms and the disease state. But such concerns have not been verified by scientific research; in fact, the opposite has been demonstrated. In one landmark study, conducted by Drs. André Dupuis, Robert Jones, and Charles Peterson, ten diabetic patients were given a standard test, the Hamilton Rating Scale. They also were interviewed by a psychiatrist. During the interview, only a few of the patients acknowledged having emotional problems; most blamed whatever problems they had on poor medical treatment and other external factors. But a much different picture emerged from evaluation of the Hamilton scores. A report published by the researchers elaborates, "They consistently felt helpless, hopeless, and worthless. A loss of self-esteem permeated their lives. Few felt that they could control their diabetes." Nine of the ten patients had higher than normal depression scores; many had difficulty functioning at work, and hypochondriasis, or preoccupation with illness and symptoms, was common.

All ten of the patients had poorly controlled diabetes. What's more, those with the poorest control had the most pronounced psychological symptoms. At the outset there had been some concern that the high degree of depression might prevent some of the patients from complying with the discipline and details involved in effective self-care.

Recognizing these potential hazards, the researchers set about teaching the patients diabetes self-care, with emphasis on monitoring of their own blood glucose. Their improved blood sugar profiles were documented by substantial lowering of hemoglobin A_{1C}, which ranged from a 6.5 to 14 percent, with a mean of 10.3 percent at the beginning of the study (3 to 6 percent is normal). After eight months of intensive self-care with physician supervision, the mean hemoglobin A_{1C} had dropped to 5.4 percent, and eight of the ten were in the normal range. Equally striking was the improvement in emotional well-being. "At the end of the eight months of observation," the researchers wrote, "the patients were by and large proud of their ability to achieve better control of their diabetes. They spontaneously verbalized their feelings of well-being and were enthusiastic about having taken control of their illness." They no longer blamed their problems on others; any remaining emotional problems were recognized as being from within. Their problems were not all solved, but all the participants were better able to function both in their jobs and personal lives, and they no longer felt hopeless or helpless.

"When self-monitoring of blood glucose first came on the scene," recalls Dr. Dupuis, a psychiatrist at Cornell University Medical College, "many doctors were concerned that it would increase rather than reduce psychological problems. Our studies have found that these fears are, for the most part, groundless. By learning to measure their own blood glucose, instead of relying on urine testing, and learning how to make the necessary adjustments to normalize blood sugar, diabetic patients are able to gain a new sense of control."

SUMMING UP

Diabetes and emotions are interrelated from a number of different aspects. The very nature of diabetes—a chronic disease that requires constant attention and that can be exacerbated by even trivial upsets and events—produces understandable negative psychological responses. In turn, these responses can themselves hinder diabetes control. It is important that diabetic patients learn how to anticipate and manage the stresses that are a normal part of living. In addition, effective diabetes self-care also has been shown to improve the mental health status of patients with previously poorly controlled diabetes.

11

Diabetes and the Eyes

People with diabetes often describe a deep, recurring fear of losing their eyesight—a fear that is well grounded since the eyes are among the many organs that can be damaged by diabetes. In fact, diabetes is the leading cause of adult blindness in this country, and after five to ten years of living with the disease, most patients have at least some evidence of eye damage. Almost every part of the eye is adversely affected by the disease, although some changes have a greater impact on sight than others. The most worrisome complications are those affecting the lens, leading to diabetic cataracts, and the retina, resulting in diabetic retinopathy. Diabetes also may cause a type of intractable glaucoma as a result of an overgrowth of the membrane covering the iris.

Unfortunately, there are still many unanswered questions about the manner in which diabetes damages eye tissue. Some researchers are convinced that excessive blood sugar is the basic problem; others feel that an additional genetic defect that is closely related to diabetes is responsible for the eye damage. Both sides can point to seemingly conflicting evidence to support their theories. Some studies, for example, have found that improved control of blood sugar leads to a reduction in eye disorders, while others have found an apparent worsening of certain eye complications among patients put on insulin pumps, despite the fact that normal glucose levels were achieved. In a recent review article on management of diabetic retinopathy, a group of researchers from Cornell and Rockefeller Universities noted, "The answer in human studies is still controversial, but the evidence is mounting to suggest that glucose plays a role in retinopathy." These researchers also cite a number of animal studies showing that both cataracts and retinopathy associated with diabetes can be prevented by maintaining normal blood glucose.

DIABETIC CATARACTS

Two types of lens abnormalities are associated with diabetes: transient alterations in the refractive power and a clouding of the lens that is indistinguishable from the cataracts commonly seen in older, nondiabetic people. Although diabetic cataracts are seemingly identical to those that are considered a normal part of aging, the problem occurs far more frequently and at an earlier age among people with diabetes. For example, a British study found that diabetic patients forty to forty-nine years old were five to seven times more likely to undergo cataract surgery than nondiabetics in the same age group. Other studies have found that cataracts mature earlier and more rapidly in people with diabetes than in the general population.

In recent years, a number of animal studies have been conducted to identify the mechanism for cataract development in diabetes. These studies, while not definitive for humans, have demonstrated that the rate of cataract formation is directly related to blood sugar levels. Conversely, researchers have shown that the incidence of cataracts among diabetic animals can be reduced by lowering blood sugar levels, either by giving insulin, by fasting, or by feeding a diet high in fats and low in carbohydrates. The precise mechanism of cataract formation is still unknown, although studies have identified specific metabolic and other changes that appear to contribute to clouding of the lens. For example, laboratory studies have shown that glucose can bind with lens crystallin proteins, a process known as glycosylation. These combined substances do not defract light properly. Eventually, they form brownish pigments that are similar to those found in cataracts. Enzyme changes associated with high blood glucose also may contribute to cellular damage to the lens.

While scientists continue to search for the process or processes that result in diabetic cataracts, it is increasingly clear that patients with diabetes can help prevent premature cataracts by working to keep their blood sugar at normal levels. It is also important to see an ophthalmologist regularly so that any eye abnormalities can be detected and treated in an early stage. In cataracts, this usually involves removal of the diseased lens and then wearing a contact lens or glasses designed to overcome the farsightedness that occurs when the natural lens is removed. In some cases, an artificial plastic lens may be placed in the eye at the time of the operation or at a future date.

DIABETIC RETINOPATHY

The retina, the layer of light-sensitive cells that lines the back three quarters of the eyeball, is particularly susceptible to damage from diabetes. Evidence of retinopathy usually begins to show up within about five years after the onset of diabetes; in five to nine years, 27 percent of all type 1 diabetics have some degree of retinopathy. The incidence increases to 71 percent in people who have had diabetes for ten or more years, and after twenty years, the incidence rises to 90 percent.

There are several types of diabetic retinopathy, most of which do not cause serious loss of vision. The most common characteristics are various abnormalities in the tiny blood vessels that nourish the retina. The capillary walls weaken and balloon out, forming many microaneurysms. Some of the blood vessels become constricted and die. If the retina does not get enough blood to supply adequate nourishment, some of the tissue will die, forming tiny areas called cotton wool exudates because of their appearance when viewed through a magnifying device. The weakened vessels also may leak blood into the retina, resulting in dot or flame hemorrhages. These hemorrhages may reduce the sharpness of vision, but do not generally cause a serious loss of sight.

A more serious cause of concern is proliferative retinopathy, the medical term used to describe the overgrowth of new blood vessels on the retina. These vessels tend to be very fragile and will leak blood into the vitreous humor, the jellylike substance that fills most of the eyeball, dimming vision or even causing temporary blindness. In time, the blood is reabsorbed and vision returns. But scar tissue may form, resulting in damage to the retina and permanent partial loss of vision. As the scar tissue spreads, it may cause the retina to become detached, which in turn can result in blindness.

In most patients, the eye complications do not reach this proliferative stage, while in others it may occur at an early age. Factors that seem to increase the likelihood of proliferative retinopathy include age of the patient and duration of the disease; the younger the onset of diabetes, the greater the chance of serious eye problems. Hypertension, smoking, pregnancy, and the presence of other complications, such as kidney disease or neuropathy, also increase the likelihood of serious retinopathy. Clotting abnormalities, particularly platelet abnormalities that may stimulate the overgrowth of new blood vessels, also are thought to contribute to retinopathy.

The question of blood glucose control is a subject of continuing debate among experts. A number of studies indicate that people whose diabetes is under good control are less likely to have serious proliferative retinopathy than those whose blood sugar tends to be abnormally high. In addition, in a number of cases bringing blood sugar down to a normal range has resulted in marked improvement in retinopathy. But there are also cases in which a rapid lowering of blood sugar has, at least temporarily, worsened the condition. To prevent this, Self-Care doctors advocate that patients with poorly controlled diabetes and proliferative retinopathy have their blood sugar lowered gradually, and extra caution be exercised to avoid episodes of hypoglycemia. During the period of gradual normalization of blood sugar, the eyes should be checked frequently for any signs of worsening of the retinopathy. Once normal blood sugar is achieved and maintained over a period of time, past experience indicates that improvement and even some reversal in the retinal disease can be expected.

TREATMENT OF RETINOPATHY

In recent years, the use of lasers—highly concentrated light beams—to treat proliferative retinopathy has saved the eyesight of many people who previously would have gone blind. The lasers can be used to block the vessels that are leaking blood into the retina and vitreous humor. They also are used to destroy tiny portions of the retina, thinning out the tissue and increasing the underlying blood flow so the retina will get more oxygen and other nutrients. Although these treatments may result in a loss of night vision and in some difficulty in focusing, they are often effective in preventing blindness. If the proliferative retinopathy recurs, the laser treatments may have to be repeated.

In some cases, at least partial eyesight can be restored by removing the vitreous humor and replacing it with an artificial substance. Advances in microsurgery also have made it possible to repair detached retinas and certain other abnormalities caused by progressive retinopathy.

Since certain other conditions, such as high blood pressure or pregnancy, tend to accelerate eye disease, extra attention aimed at prevention is called for. Control of high blood pressure is important to prevent heart attacks, strokes, and kidney failure and also to prevent eye complications. During pregnancy, a woman should see her ophthalmologist regularly and be particularly attuned to any changes in vision. Not smoking—an important health benefit for everyone—is even more crucial for people with diabetes. Smoking has a profound effect on circulation, platelet abnormalities, and other factors thought to contribute to retinopathy; not smoking not only lowers this risk, but also reduces the risk of heart attacks and other life-threatening disorders, which already is increased by diabetes.

SUMMING UP

Diabetes is the leading cause of adult blindness in this country. Although many questions about the relationship of diabetes and eye disease remain unanswered, there is growing evidence that maintaining normal blood glucose may prevent many cases of diabetic cataracts and retinopathy. Advanced methods of treatment using lasers and microsurgery also are improving the outlook for many diabetic patients with serious eye disease.

12

Diabetes and the Cardiovascular System

People with diabetes have a much higher incidence of circulatory disorders than the general population. These problems affect both the large blood vessels, such as the coronary arteries, which nourish the heart, and the carotid artery, which carries blood to the brain, and the microcirculation, which includes the tiny blood vessels of the eye. The end results of these circulatory problems are diverse: not only do people with diabetes have more heart attacks and strokes, they also are more likely to have impaired circulation, especially in the hands and feet, leading to gangrene and limb amputations.

Diabetic patients also tend to have high blood pressure and elevated blood lipids (cholesterol and triglycerides)—two factors that are known to increase the risk of heart attacks and strokes. Arteriosclerosis, or hardening of the arteries, appears to begin at an earlier age and advance more rapidly in people with diabetes: diabetic patients have a twofold increase in arteriosclerotic heart disease that is not explained by other cardiovascular risk factors. Before the discovery of insulin, the cardiovascular complications of diabetes were not so evident since so many people with the disease succumbed to diabetic coma or other primary complications. But autopsy studies performed in the 1920s and 1930s clearly established the high incidence of advanced cardiovascular disease among diabetics who were still relatively young. Women, who ordinarily have a lower incidence of heart attacks than men until they reach menopause, appear to be particularly vulnerable to the elevated blood cholesterol and triglyceride level that often accompanies diabetes.

A number of studies have documented that about half of all deaths in the United States are caused by arteriosclerosis, but the risk is doubled in men with diabetes and increased four- to sixfold in diabetic women. In all, about three fourths of all deaths in diabetic patients are caused by arteriosclerotic complications. This is reflected in the Diabetes Self-Care Program's extra effort to reduce cardiovascular risk factors in addition to controlling blood glucose. Specifically, attempts are made to control high blood pressure, eliminate cigarette smoking, and lower high cholesterol. All of these factors have been shown to greatly increase the chances of a heart attack; the more risk factors that are present, the greater the likelihood of dying from cardiovascular disease.

Although most experts agree that diabetic patients should make a special effort to reduce cardiovascular risk factors, the coronary disease that occurs with diabetes is somewhat different from that in the general population. This point was emphasized by Dr. W. Virgil Brown, a noted New York cardiologist, at a recent conference on diabetes management held under the direction of Dr. Peterson at Rockefeller University. At that meeting, Dr. Brown summarized these major differences:

• Diabetic patients have a much higher cardiovascular death rate and they also are less likely to survive a heart attack than are nondiabetics.

• Silent or undiagnosed heart attacks are more common among people with diabetes.

• The coronary arteries of diabetic patients are more diseased than those of nondiabetics, and the nature of the disease is somewhat different. The fatty deposits (atheromas) not only are more extensive, they also contain larger quantities of calcium and other materials.

• Disease of the heart muscle itself is more common among diabetic patients, leading to an increased risk of heart failure and other cardiac abnormalities.

The reasons for these differences are unknown, although the following possible explanations are under study.

Lipid Abnormalities

Diabetic patients are particularly apt to have unfavorable lipoprotein ratios (see page 123). In recent years, increasing attention has been paid not only to lowering total cholesterol, but also to achieving a higher ratio of HDL compared to LDL. The Framingham Heart Study—the longest and most comprehensive epidemiological research project ever undertaken in this country—has followed the residents of this Boston suburb for four decades and has clearly demonstrated that a high level of LDL and low HDL increases the risk of a heart attack. This study has also found that women with diabetes tend to have greatly reduced HDL, which may explain their higher incidence of cardiovascular disease. Other epidemiological studies have found that diabetic populations with low LDL levels also have a low incidence of cardiovascular disease. Thus, as noted by Dr. Brown at the Rockefeller conference on diabetes, "LDL deserves attention as a very powerful risk factor in all individuals, including diabetics."

A number of factors have been identified that improve the HDL-LDL ratio. Perhaps most important for diabetic patients are recent studies indicating that maintenance of normal blood glucose appears to increase HDL levels. Other factors that improve the HDL-LDL ratio include physical activity—people who exercise regularly have higher HDL—and a diet low in cholesterol and saturated fats. Since the recommended diabetes diet tends to be higher in total fat than that urged for the general population, people with the disease need to pay particular attention to the types of fat they consume. Polyunsaturated fats, which are found in vegetable oils (except palm and coconut) and some fish, tend to lower cholesterol, while saturated fats (animal fats, coconut and palm oils, and oils that have been hardened to maintain a solid form at room temperature) raise it. A diet high in cholesterol, which is found in animal fats and dairy products, particularly whole milk, butter, cheese, and egg yolks, also raise LDL cholesterol. Thus, people with diabetes should take care that their diets emphasize polyunsaturated fats in preference to saturated fats and foods high in cholesterol. (See Chapter 6 for a more complete discussion.)

Obesity is also a factor in elevated blood lipids and cardiovascular disease. People who are overweight tend to have high blood cholesterol. Weight gain also raises triglyceride levels. In addition, the Framingham Study has identified obesity as still another factor increasing the risk of a heart attack. Since most people with type 2 diabetes tend to be overweight, maintaining ideal weight is doubly important for these patients, not only in controlling diabetes but also as a possible preventive of heart disease.

Hypertension

A number of studies have confirmed that people with diabetes are more likely to develop high blood pressure than the nondiabetic population. One study, for example, found that half of the patients surveyed who had had diabetes for thirty or more years also had high blood pressure. As noted earlier, this is reflected in the increased risk of heart attacks among diabetic patients. High blood pressure is the major cause of strokes. It is also a significant factor in kidney disease and exacerbates the eye problems that so often afflict people with diabetes.

Several major epidemiological studies, including Framingham, have found that diabetic women seem to have a higher prevalence of hypertension than men. In any event, the hypertension should be controlled since it is an additional risk factor for heart attacks, strokes, kidney failure, blindness, problems during pregnancy, and other serious disorders. There are now a number of drugs that are highly effective in lowering high blood pressure. Restricting salt, maintaining normal weight, avoiding unnecessary stress, and exercising are also important elements in controlling blood pressure.

Platelet Abnormalities

Platelets are the blood components responsible for clotting. A number of researchers have linked platelet abnormalities with increased atherosclerosis, the buildup of fatty deposits in the arteries. The exact mechanism remains unknown, but one possible theory goes like this: The cells that line the blood vessels, the endothelium, are injured, perhaps by the biochemical abnormalities associated with diabetes, by a viral infection, or by the extra stress on the arteries caused by high blood pressure. This injury stimulates the platelets to clump, or aggregate, at the site. The clumping platelets produce a chemical called thromboxane, which causes further aggregation and stickiness of the platelets, as well as a narrowing or constriction of the blood vessel. This increases blood pressure and may further injure the endothelial tissue, which in turn produces further platelet clumping. Eventually fatty streaks appear along the vessel wall, which progress to the artery-narrowing atheromas that are characteristic of progressive atherosclerosis. If the affected vessel is a coronary artery, a portion of the heart muscle may not get enough oxygen, especially when the heart's workload is increased. This may result in angina pectoris, the temporary chest pains that signal coronary disease. The vessel may become totally blocked by the fatty plaque or by a blood clot (a coronary thrombosis), resulting in a heart attack.

Abnormal Red Blood Cells

Oxygen is carried through the body via hemoglobin, a component of red blood cells. A number of diseases are characterized by abnormalities in these important blood cells. For example, iron deficiency reduces the amount of hemoglobin in the blood, resulting in anemia. Abnormal development of red blood cells, such as might occur in sickle-cell anemia or some types of blood cancer, also limits the blood's ability to deliver oxygen to body tissues. In diabetes, high blood sugar has a marked effect on hemoglobin and oxygen delivery. Some of the glucose molecules attach themselves to the hemoglobin, changing their structure. The combined molecules, known as hemoglobin A_{1C} or glycosylated hemoglobin, does not carry as much oxygen as normal hemoglobin, thereby further impairing the body's circulatory system. By measuring the level of glycosylated hemoglobin, physicians can determine the degree of blood sugar control over a period of time. For example, a 10 percent hemoglobin A_{1C} indicates that the mean blood glucose for the preceding month or so has been about 200 mg/dl.

Studies also have found that the red blood cells age more rapidly in diabetic patients. The increased turnover of red blood cells puts an added burden on the circulatory system.

Abnormalities of Capillaries

So far we have concentrated on diabetes-caused abnormalities in the arteries; however, the disease also affects the microcirculation, or the tiny capillaries that provide blood for the individual body cells. In diabetes, there is a thickening of the basement membranes, the substance that separates the epithelial cells that line the various body surfaces from the underlying structures. A thickening of the capillary basement membranes alters the blood vessels' blood-carrying function, resulting in a reduction in the amount of blood that is delivered to the body tissues.

Insulin

Researchers have long been concerned that insulin itself may play a role in promoting atherosclerosis. Laboratory studies have found that insulin can increase lipid synthesis within the artery walls, which may promote the buildup of fatty streaks—the forerunner of atherosclerosis. Many people with type 2 diabetes have higher than normal levels of insulin, which their bodies fail to use effectively. Other studies have found that insulin can increase proliferation of smooth muscle cells, which may further affect the artery walls. A number of laboratory studies have suggested that an overgrowth of muscle cells is one of the early stages of arteriosclerosis. But it has not been proved that this is an outcome of diabetes. Nor is there definitive evidence that the insulin taken to control diabetes leads to arterial disease.

OTHER CIRCULATORY DISORDERS

Of course, the increased vascular disease is not limited to the coronary arteries; other blood vessels also are adversely affected. Poor circulation to the lower limbs is particularly common, leading to a loss of sensation, chronic skin ulcers, pain, and, in extreme cases, gangrene and amputation. The reduced blood flow and progressive hardening of arteries may result in a condition called intermittent claudication—a disorder that produces severe pain and disability. People with intermittent claudication may be seriously limited in their ability to walk, climb stairs, or use their legs. The disorder also may cause severe cramping or pain even when resting, resulting in disrupted sleep. Some studies, such as a large-scale epidemiological project in Tecumseh, Michigan, have correlated severe intermittent claudication with poorly controlled blood sugar. The Framingham Study has found that diabetic women are affected more commonly than men and that smoking increases the problem significantly. As might be expected, high blood pressure also seems to worsen the vascular disease and increase the risk of gangrene and amputation.

People with diabetes should be particularly careful to avoid infections and injuries in the lower limbs and feet (see Chapter 18). Avoiding smoking and getting regular exercise also are important preventive measures. Reducing other risk factors, such as lowering high blood pressure and keeping blood cholesterol in check, may minimize the problems associated with diabetic vascular disease.

THE RISK OF STROKES

Stroke, or cerebrovascular accident, is an area that is often overlooked in discussing circulatory problems associated with diabetes. However, studies in both Israel and Framingham have found that people with diabetes have a twofold increase in strokes. Little is known about any link between diabetes and strokes, but since high blood pressure is known to be the major cause of strokes, and diabetic patients have a higher than normal incidence of hypertension, it seems logical that controlling blood pressure is a major factor in stroke prevention.

SUMMING UP

Arteriosclerosis is the major cause of death and disability among people with diabetes. A number of factors are involved, including high blood pressure, elevated blood lipids, obesity, and cigarette smoking. But it is not known if or how diabetes itself increases the risk of vascular disease. At present, most experts, including doctors with the Diabetes Self-Care Program, advocate that diabetic patients be particularly diligent about reducing as many of the controllable cardiovascular risk factors as possible. This includes paying close attention to diet to keep cholesterol and other blood lipids low, reducing high blood pressure, maintaining ideal weight, exercising, and not smoking.

13

Diabetic Neuropathy

Diabetes is a disease that affects almost every body system. In the nervous system this leads to a host of complications known as diabetic neuropathy. These complications may manifest themselves in a number of ways: loss of sensation and nervous function, intermittent episodes of pain, slowed reflexes, coordination problems, and sexual impotence in men are among the many signs of neuropathy.

In the early stages of diabetic neuropathy, there may be no obvious symptoms. But as the disorder progresses, symptoms such as tingling sensations in the fingers and toes, muscular weakness or a loss of feeling, especially in the lower limbs, may become apparent. Diabetic neuropathy is an important factor in the foot ulcerations and other problems experienced by many patients. If the neuropathy dulls the pain sensation, the person may be unaware that he or she has developed a blister, corn, callus, or other problem until a serious infection occurs. Since diabetes interferes with the body's natural defenses against infection and the disease also may reduce the flow of blood to the affected area, something that ordinarily would be a minor injury that would quickly heal instead becomes a major infection that can threaten the entire limb.

Pain is a common feature of diabetic neuropathy. In some patients, the pain is limited to a mild discomfort or tingling sensations, while others suffer from severe, disabling pain. Some people have excessively sensitive skin; even the slightest touch will produce severe pain. Others experience shooting or stabbing pains that come and go without apparent cause. Still others describe a bone-deep aching pain that may make sleep impossible. A number of different factors may be involved in causing the pain associated with diabetic neuropathy. For example, some neurologists suggest that destruction of some of the large nerve fibers, which are thought to be important in suppressing pain sensations, may be a factor. Or a regeneration of small nerve fibers may produce pain, especially in the skin.

Until recently, most diabetes experts assumed that diabetic neuropathy was a late complication of long-standing, poorly controlled disease. This assumption has been disproved with the development of more sophisticated tests of nerve function and health. It is now known that nerve deterioration may begin in the early stages of diabetics and affects both motor (nerves that carry impulses to the muscles and are instrumental in movement) and sensory (nerves that carry sensations of pain, hot, cold, and other feelings) functions, even though the symptoms may not become apparent for many years. The problem occurs in both type 1 and type 2 diabetes.

It had also been assumed that the legs were affected more than the arms and other body parts. This, too, has been disproved by researchers using new nerve-function tests. These studies have found that although the legs may seem to suffer greater nerve disease, the arms are equally affected—the difference is in the degree of obvious symptoms. Also, not everyone experiences symptoms. Some diabetic patients can have widespread neuropathy and experience only minor symptoms, while others will experience a variety of problems that become progressively worse. Some patients, for example, develop muscular weakness and wasting (atrophy), while others may have advanced neuropathy with little obvious effects on the muscles.

The autonomic nervous system, which controls the working of organs and processes over which we have no direct control (e.g., the cardiovascular or digestive systems), has not been studied as extensively as other types of neuropathy, but it also is affected by diabetes. Sexual impotence is one of the more common manifestations of neuropathy affecting the autonomic nervous systems. Others include gastrointestinal problems, bladder disorders, irregular heartbeats, or blood pressure abnormalities, such as dizziness or fainting upon standing up (orthostatic hypotension). Studies have found a higher incidence of cardiac arrest and sudden death among diabetic patients with autonomic neuropathy.

POSSIBLE CAUSES OF NEUROPATHY

A number of theories regarding the underlying mechanism of diabetic neuropathy are being studied. At one time, researchers thought that most of the nerve damage occurred in the myelin—a protein substance that is produced in bodies known as Schwann cells and encases the large nerve fibers. Recent studies have found, however, that the axons—the long nerve cells that conduct impulses or messages—also are involved, perhaps even before the deterioration in the myelin. While the exact causes for the breakdown in these nerve cells are still unknown, there is considerable evidence supporting several theories, leading many experts to believe that more than one or two factors may be involved. The changes in metabolism and body chemistry that accompany diabetes are thought to be at least partly responsible for the nerve disorders. At a recent Rockefeller University conference on diabetes management, a group of University of Washington researchers summarized the following changes:

Effects of High Blood Glucose

A swelling, or buildup of fluid, between the nerve Schwann cells and axons has been observed. Some researchers theorize that this swelling is due to the metabolic abnormalities caused by hyperglycemia. They think that a complicated process involving the conversion of several different sugars into their corresponding sugar alcohols; for example, glucose into sorbitol, may be responsible.

A second theory also involving abnormal glucose metabolism suggests that hyperglycemia may cause a deficiency of myo-inositol, a vitamin in the B complex that resembles a sugar and is necessary for proper membrane function, including nerve membranes. Researchers think that hyperglycemia may interfere with the transport of this substance to the nerves, and instead, it is excreted in the urine. Studies involving laboratory animals have found that nerve function may be improved by increasing the myo-inositol content of the diet. Similarly, studies in humans have found that increasing myo-inositol intake may improve sensory nerve function in diabetic patients, but no effect was found on motor nerves. (Although these findings are encouraging, there is no evidence at present that vitamin or dietary supplements are an effective treatment for diabetic neuropathy.)

Still another theory involves alteration of nerve cells due to high blood glucose. Recent studies have found that glucose molecules attach themselves to nerve proteins, altering their structure in a manner similar to the glycosylation of red blood cells. This glycosylation of nerve cells may interfere with their ability to function normally and explain the damage to the various nerve structures.

Effects of Insulin Deficiency

A number of recent studies have shed new light on the possible role of insulin in nerve function. Researchers have found that insulin can reverse a defect in production of myelin among diabetic laboratory animals. Recent studies also have found that some central neurons have insulin receptors, indicating the hormone may have an as yet unidentified role in nerve function. If these preliminary findings turn out to be true in humans, then a lack of sufficient insulin may cause diabetic neuropathy.

Other Possible Unidentified Factors

Some researchers speculate that there is some other basic defect leading to diabetic neuropathy that is not necessarily associated with either high blood glucose or insulin deficiency. These researchers suggest that the unidentified causative factor behind neuropathy may be the same factor that leads to the breakdown in the pancreas's ability to produce insulin. As basis for this theory, these researchers cite the fact that neuropathy is often evident before there is an elevation in blood glucose and that serious nerve disease sometimes occurs before any other symptoms of diabetes.

TREATMENT OF DIABETIC NEUROPATHY

In the past, the outlook for treating diabetic neuropathy has been rather gloomy. Most doctors have assumed that the loss of nerve function was permanent and that not much could be done to prevent it from occurring. This outlook is changing in light of recent studies comparing the degree of neuropathy in patients whose diabetes is well controlled with those with consistently high blood sugar. For example, a group of British researchers recently reported the results of a two-year study involving seventy-four diabetic patients who were randomly divided into two groups. All were type 1 diabetics and all had evidence of diabetic retinopathy. One group was put on an intensive regimen that included multiple daily insulin injections, frequent visits to a diabetes clinic, dietary counseling, and self-monitoring of their own blood glucose. The second group continued their regular regimens, which were typical of diabetes treatment recommended for the general population. At the end of two years, patients in the two groups were compared for a number of complications.

Patients in the intensively treated group had lower blood glucose levels than those who continued their regular treatments, although toward the end of the study, the latter group also began to achieve lower blood sugar. In assessing diabetes complications, the researchers found that the intensively treated patients had better sensory nerve functions and also less evidence of kidney disease. They also achieved significantly lower levels of LDL cholesterol. There were no major differences, however, in eye disorders. The researchers concluded that "deterioration of nerve and renal function can be prevented by more intensive diabetic management. . . ."

This conclusion is being echoed by a growing number of diabetes experts as well as neurologists. Self-Care Program physicians, for example, stress that achieving as normal a blood sugar profile as possible offers the best hope of preventing or minimizing diabetic neuropathy. In a recent paper published in the *Annals of Neurology*, Drs. M. J. Brown and A. K. Asbury, two neurologists at the University of Pennsylvania, advised, "Because the severity of diabetic neuropathy appears to be correlated with the magnitude and duration of hyperglycemia, one should try to obtain a high degree of blood glucose control." They also noted that "the most important step in reducing pain from diabetic neuropathy may be to improve blood glucose control."

Some of the symptoms or results of diabetic neuropathy can be relieved by treatments directed specifically to them, even though they may not affect the underlying cause or the diabetes itself. For example, patients with diabetic neuropathy are urged to pay meticulous attention to skin care. This may involve inspecting the feet and hands a couple of times a day to make sure that there are no unnoticed injuries that may develop into serious infections. Any break in the skin or sign of inflammation requires prompt treatment. Painkillers and other drugs may provide some relief for pain associated with neuropathy, but the type of drug and dosage should be determined by a doctor. Elastic stockings and drugs may help relieve the orthostatic hypotension related to neuropathy of the autonomic system. Footdrop or ankle weakness may be relieved by braces or other mechanical devices.

Impotence is understandably a highly troublesome complication for many diabetic men. Unfortunately, many men are embarrassed or reluctant to discuss sexual difficulties with their doctors or even their sexual partners. The impotence associated with diabetes usually is organic rather than psychological. The problem may involve inability to achieve or maintain an erection or abnormalities of ejaculation. Recent advances in devices that are implanted in the penis to help achieve an erection may help many patients suffering from impotence regain their ability to have sexual intercourse. Several types of penile prostheses have been developed; some are of a rigid construction while others are inflatable. Information about these prostheses can be obtained from urologists who are experienced in treating sexual problems in diabetic men.

Summing Up

Neuropathy is a very common complication of diabetes. Although it does not always produce noticeable symptoms, especially in the early stages of the disease, sophisticated nerve studies have found that most people with either type of diabetes have some evidence of nerve deterioration. The cause or causes of diabetic neuropathy are unknown, although there is evidence that high blood glucose or a lack of insulin may be important factors. A number of studies have found that patients with poorly controlled diabetes are more apt to have progressive neuropathy. By the same token, studies have found that patients whose blood sugar is well controlled are less likely to experience symptoms of neuropathy.

At present, the best approach for minimizing diabetic neuropathy seems to be maintaining tight control of blood sugar. While this does not seem to prevent the problem, it has been shown to reduce the development of overt symptoms, such as pain and muscular weakness and wasting. If symptoms do develop, relief may be obtained by a variety of treatments directed to them.

14

Diabetes and the Kidneys

Long-standing diabetes has a profound effect on the kidneys, especially if blood glucose has been consistently above normal. In poorly controlled type 1 diabetes, about 45 percent of the patients develop kidney failure within twenty-five years. Advances in treating kidney failure, especially development of hemodialysis using an artificial kidney and replacement of diseased kidneys with healthy transplants, have helped prolong the lives of these patients. They do not, however, cure the disease. Studies have found that healthy kidneys transplanted into diabetic patients develop signs of disease (diabetic nephropathy) within two to four years; similar findings have been produced in animal studies.

The kidneys are particularly vulnerable to diabetes for several reasons. Blood constantly flows through the kidneys, which, along with the lungs, filter out waste material for disposal from the body. Each kidney contains more than a million minute filtering units called nephrons. Each nephron consists of a filter, a glomerulus, which separates the liquid containing both nutrients and chemical waste material, mostly the by-products of metabolism by the cells, from the blood. The nephrons also contain long, thin tubes, called tubules, that go from the glomeruli to the medulla, or core of the kidney. The tubules are surrounded by tiny blood vessels that reabsorb the nutrients; the blood then leaves the kidney via the renal vein and returns to the general circulation. The remaining liquid containing the waste material passes into the ureter, a tube that carries it out of the kidney and to the bladder for eventual excretion from the body as urine.

This is a highly simplified explanation of how the kidneys work; they are actually highly complex, amazingly efficient organs that are essential to maintaining life. Fortunately, kidneys come in pairs; if something happens to one, the remaining organ can take over and the person can get along quite nicely. In diabetes, however, the disease usually affects both organs equally, making kidney failure a common cause of illness and death.

Excessive blood glucose is the culprit in most cases of diabetic kidney failure. Although the nephrons are extraordinarily efficient filters, there is a limit to how much glucose they can handle. The excess that cannot be reabsorbed in the tubules is excreted in the urine (glycosuria), explaining why sugary urine is a classic sign of diabetes. The high level of blood glucose causes structural changes in the nephrons; these changes include a membrane thickening that reduces their filtering capacity. Since diabetes itself increases the workload of the kidneys, any reduction in their filtering capacity results in a vicious cycle of more work and reduced ability to perform it. This is manifested not only by the presence of sugar in the urine, but also protein and other important nutrients.

Diabetes also makes the kidneys and other parts of the urinary tract more susceptible to infection, which can have a destructive effect on the kidney. People with diabetes should be particularly aware of the signs of urinary tract infections—feelings of urgency, difficulty in voiding, pain or burning sensations accompanying urination, or blood in the urine—and see a doctor promptly if they occur.

Treatment of Diabetic Nephropathy

At one time, doctors assumed that little could be done to prevent diabetic destruction of the kidneys. A number of recent studies, however, show that it may be possible to both prevent and perhaps even reverse the destructive changes in the nephron by maintaining normal blood sugar levels. Researchers at the University of Minnesota, for example, have conducted a number of pioneering studies in this area. These researchers have conducted studies in both humans and laboratory animals to determine whether the kidney damage of diabetes can be prevented or altered. They have found that tight control of the disease reduces the kidney damage, and further, that undertaking a treatment program that normalizes blood glucose can, at least in laboratory animals, reverse some of the damage from diabetes. What's more, even though the glomeruli and other nephron structures may not return to their prediabetic state, the remaining damage does not seem to alter their ability to function enough to prevent kidney failure.

Timing seems to be an important factor in the kidney's ability to recover from the damage of diabetes. The Minnesota researchers found, for example, that if diabetes is brought under tight control early in the course of the disease, the characteristic changes in the nephron may be prevented. They have also found that if effective blood sugar control is instituted before advanced kidney failure occurs, some of the damage to the nephron may be reversed. These findings have been confirmed both by kidney biopsies in human transplant patients as well as in animal studies. In reporting their findings at the Rockefeller University conference on diabetes management, the Minnesota researchers concluded, "It is clear that precise control of the diabetic state decreases the risk of [renal] complications."

Summing Up

Kidney failure has long been a major cause of death and illness among diabetic patients. Recent studies have shown that maintaining normal blood sugar may prevent much of this kidney damage, and in patients who already show signs of kidney disease, instituting a program of tight control may reverse some of the damage.

15

Diabetes and the Risk of Infection

Infections of all kinds pose a special threat to the person with diabetes. From time to time, virtually everyone suffers a cold or other viral illness, infected cut, bout of cystitis, annoying fungal infection, or some other ordinarily trivial infectious disorder. After a few days of making us feel miserable, the problem usually disappears, often without any treatment or with the help of an antibiotic or other appropriate medication. For the person with diabetes, however, a common infection can become a major problem, leading to difficulty in controlling blood sugar and in overcoming the infection. At the first sign of illness, even the onset of a common cold, you should contact your doctor. This is particularly important if a bacterial infection may be involved, because the earlier the invading organism can be identified and treatment started with the right antibiotic, the better the chances of cure without complications.

Insulin resistance is one of the early consequences of infection in the diabetic person. In fact, blood sugar often rises before symptoms of infection become apparent. This is part of the body's complex hormonal and metabolic responses to infection. These responses and the increased insulin resistance may be further complicated by the fact that the infection itself may affect appetite and food intake. For example, nausea, vomiting, or diarrhea often accompany an infection. These complications may make blood glucose control even more difficult. Ordinarily, if you are unable to eat, you usually must lower insulin accordingly. But during an infection, the body usually needs more insulin, so a lowering of insulin dosage may not be appropriate.

Physical activity also may be lowered, resulting in reduced burning of glucose. All these factors may lead to a rapid rise in blood sugar and the development of ketoacidosis. Of course, there is also a danger of overcompensating and taking more insulin than the body can handle, leading to serious hypoglycemia and even coma. This is why self-monitoring of both blood sugar and the urine for signs of ketones and being particularly sensitive to any symptoms of hypoglycemia are so important during any infection or illness. In fact, if you have even the slightest doubts about being able to maintain control, you should seek help without delay. This may even mean checking into a hospital until the infection is under control and the diabetes is again in check.

DIABETES AND THE IMMUNE SYSTEM

People with diabetes not only have increased difficulty in overcoming an infection, they also are more vulnerable to developing infectious disorders because the disease lowers the body's natural resistance. How diabetes affects the body's immune system is not fully understood; the disease itself is thought to be caused, at least in part, by defects in the immune system. Type 1 diabetes often develops soon after a viral infection, and people with the disease also tend to produce antibodies against parts of their own body, in particular the insulin-producing structures in the islets of Langerhans. Thus, some sort of genetic defect in the immune system may be responsible for causing diabetes.

As the disease develops, the body's natural defenses are further affected. Studies by Dr. Peterson and his Rockefeller University colleagues have found that poorly controlled diabetes interferes with the ability of the white blood cells (leukocytes) to fight invading bacteria and other microorganisms. This lowering in the body's natural defense system makes diabetic patients highly susceptible to a variety of infections, including from organisms that ordinarily may inhabit the body or environment without causing illness. Diseases caused by these normally benign organisms in people with faulty immune systems are referred to as opportunistic infections, and they often involve fungi or ordinarily harmless bacteria.

Types of infections that are particularly common among people with diabetes include urinary tract infections; thrush, periodontal disease, and other mouth infections; and wound infections of all kinds. The feet and hands, which frequently have impaired circulation and nerve function caused by diabetes, are particularly vulnerable. Even the slightest cut or blister can develop into a chronic ulcer and even gangrene. Since the feeling of pain is often reduced by diabetic neuropathy, people with diabetes should be particularly careful to avoid wound infections, including those that may develop at insulin injection sites. Special care should be taken to observe good hygiene and sterile practices; any sign of inflammation—for example, a tender, reddened area around the site of infusion from an insulin pump—should be seen by a doctor without delay.

Women with diabetes are particularly susceptible to yeast and other vaginal infections. These infections are best eradicated when the glucose level is normalized. This infection per se usually does not affect the insulin requirement. Many doctors advise these women not to use tampons, particularly the superabsorbant kind that have been linked to an increased risk of toxic shock syndrome, a serious blood infection caused by a staphylococcus organism. Vaginal and urinary tract infections may be particularly troublesome during pregnancy, which in itself increases their likelihood. Urinary tract infection, on the other hand, does increase insulin requirements and should be treated promptly to avoid a retrograde infection to the kidneys.

PREVENTION OF INFECTION

Some infective illnesses are virtually unavoidable, but many others can be prevented, either by practicing good general hygiene or by specific measures, such as immunization. Diabetic patients are among the high-risk groups that should have periodic immunization against influenza and bacterial pneumonia.

In a more general sense, achieving good blood glucose control also helps prevent infectious disorders. Studies have found that when normal blood sugar levels are achieved, the body's defense system is also strengthened. White blood cells return to normal and are able to better overcome infection. Other complications that predispose the diabetic patient to infection, such as impaired circulation and neuropathy, also may improve under good glucose control, thereby reducing the risk of infection.

Extra precautions to prevent infections may be required during pregnancy. People undergoing surgery or even routine dental work also may require special preventive measures, such as taking a broad-spectrum antibiotic. Any injury, no matter how minor, requires extra attention. Fortunately, the development of effective antibiotics has helped reduce the life-threatening aspects of many infections, but early treatment remains a vital component in the total approach to treating diabetes.

SUMMING UP

Infections are doubly troublesome for people with diabetes. These illnesses not only make blood sugar more difficult to control by increasing insulin resistance, they also may prove difficult to treat because of lowered resistance and diabetes-related changes in the immune system. Other complications of diabetes, such as impaired blood circulation, kidney disease, and nerve disorders, also may increase the risk of infection and make it more difficult to treat.

Early recognition and treatment of any infection is particularly important for diabetic patients. Prevention of infection is also an important aspect of the total treatment of diabetes. This includes undergoing appropriate immunizations, practicing good hygiene, and, perhaps most important, achieving good blood glucose control, a factor that has been shown to bolster the body's natural defenses against infection.

III

Problem Solving

16

Diabetes in Childhood

Type 1 diabetes often first appears during childhood or adolescence. Before the discovery of insulin, most children who contracted the disease had little hope of reaching adulthood. Today the majority of diabetic children not only grow up, they also can lead healthy, relatively normal lives. But there are often many difficulties along the way, both medical and emotional.

Diabetes is a difficult disease for the entire family, and designing an effective treatment program often means counseling each member. Diabetes Self-Care Program physicians repeatedly emphasize that controlling the disease goes beyond insulin dosages, diet, and exercise —the stresses of day-to-day life also are crucial in keeping blood glucose in check. The attitudes of parents, siblings, and even friends are important factors; creating a normal environment for healthy development and at the same time managing a difficult disease that needs constant attention are major challenges for everyone involved. The diabetic child must be made to understand that he or she has a serious disease that requires constant treatment and monitoring, but at the same time the youngster should know that he or she is not an invalid; normal activities are not only possible, they are a desirable part of the overall therapy. From the outset, it is important to establish a good rapport with a physician who will oversee the treatment. This doctor should be someone experienced in treating diabetic children and someone that both the patient and parents can relate to. Many doctors are attuned to treating a series of short-term crises; diabetes, however, is lifelong. Although the patient or, in the case of a young child, the parent carries on the day-to-day control of the disease, the doctor must be available not only to lend support and information but to handle any difficult situations that might arise.

Aside from the misfortune of contracting a chronic disease at an early age, childhood diabetes poses a different spectrum of treatment problems. The amount of insulin required may be difficult to gauge. The frequent viral infections that are common in early childhood affect the amount of insulin needed. Growth also alters insulin needs: the dosage usually rises sharply during growth spurts. In addition, the lifestyle of a normal, active child often is contrary to what is needed to maintain good blood sugar control. Most youngsters, for example, tend to be emotionally labile—sunny one moment and in tears or a state of temper the next. Maintaining a regular schedule of food intake and exercise are contrary to the way most children behave: they exercise in spurts, and when they are hungry they usually will wolf down whatever is handy. The trick is to find a middle ground that does not hamper normal development but is still in keeping with the treatment program.

The disease also puts a tremendous strain on other family members. Siblings may resent the extra attention that is given the diabetic child. Parents are often filled with guilt, anxiety, or worry—emotions that are quickly communicated to the child. "Treating the child with diabetes usually means working with the entire family," says Dr. Jovanovic, "at least in the beginning."

Childhood onset of diabetes often follows a period of stress, frequently a viral illness. An emotional upheaval—divorce or loss of a parent or some other major change—may bring on the first obvious symptoms, as may the growth spurt and hormonal changes of puberty. The precise relationship of these stresses to diabetes onset is unknown, but often parents feel they somehow could have prevented the disease if they had acted differently, resulting in misplaced feelings of guilt. No one knows how to prevent diabetes, and a child's contracting it is no one's fault. Most researchers believe that a combination of genetic and environmental factors are involved, but no one knows precisely what these are. Self-Care physicians take special pains to help parents understand that they are not to blame for their child's diabetes.

The symptoms of diabetes in a child are similar to those in an older person, but they may appear more rapidly, sometimes in a matter of hours or a few days. These symptoms include excessive thirst and urination; usually the child has to get up several times during the night to urinate or may wet the bed. There also may be a rapid loss of weight despite a voracious appetite and eating more than normal. Such symptoms should alert a parent to take the child to a doctor promptly, since ketoacidosis and diabetic coma may develop quickly. The initial onset is often followed by a "honeymoon phase," a period of remission that may last for only a few weeks up to several months or even longer. During this period, the failing pancreas strives to increase its insulin output. Little or no insulin may be needed, but the child should be carefully observed for a recurrence of symptoms and monitored frequently for a telltale rise in blood sugar, which signals advancing failure of the pancreas to produce insulin.

TREATING CHILDHOOD DIABETES

Treating childhood diabetes is perhaps even more of a team effort than controlling the disease in an older person. Very often, the treatment program is developed in a hospital setting. The child may have to be hospitalized to overcome ketoacidosis and to stabilize blood sugar. The hospital period also gives doctors, dietitians, and other health professionals a chance to teach both the parents and patient about the disease. In very young children, the burden of care and monitoring falls on the parents. Many young children are terrified of getting injections, and the idea of having two or three a day adds to their understandable anxiety. Parents also may be frightened at the prospect of administering injections, especially if they have never done it before. There is also the negative connotation of associating hypodermic needles with illicit drug use; children, especially those who have been exposed to drug education programs in school and elsewhere, should be reassured that their injections are in no way associated with street drugs and addicts. Fortunately, the fears and apprehensions surrounding injections are quickly overcome when they become a part of the daily routine. As soon as possible, children should be taught how to manage their diabetes. Generally, children can begin to administer their own injections by the time they are seven or eight years old, although parental reminding may be needed. By the age of eight or so, most children also can learn the basics of self-monitoring.

In the past, many doctors treating diabetic children did not attempt to maintain normal glucose. Before self-testing of blood glucose became possible, urine testing was the only available yardstick for monitoring glucose, and it is not reliable. Since episodes of hypoglycemia are a particular worry in managing childhood diabetes, there was a tendency to undertreat; in other words, to strive for an insulin dosage sufficient to prevent the ketoacidosis that may occur from very high blood sugar, but not necessarily enough to normalize glucose levels. "The idea was to get a child or adolescent through the growing phase, and then to try to establish tighter control in young adulthood," Dr. Peterson explains. "Of course, the problem with this approach is that by the time the child grows up, there already may be severe kidney disease, eye damage, or other serious complications." It is well established that the most severe diabetic complications occur in patients who developed the disease at an early age. "Despite the difficulties involved in maintaining good glucose control in a child," Dr. Peterson adds, "we have good reason to believe that this will help prevent later long-term complications."

The Value of Home Glucose Monitoring

Until now, we have concentrated on the role of self-testing of blood sugar in adults; the Self-Care Program also advocates this important tool in treating the diabetic child. At a recent Rockefeller University conference on diabetes management, an Australian researcher, Dr. M. Selink of the Royal Alexander Hospital for Children in Camperdown, reported the results of a study to evaluate home blood glucose testing in fifty children. The youngsters ranged from four to eighteen years of age and were selected because "they were the most difficult to stabilize using standard urine testing or because of a tendency to have unpredictable hypoglycemic episodes. . . . Thus they represented the more difficult end of the spectrum of childhood diabetes." There were twenty-eight boys and twenty-two girls in the study; the mean ages were eleven and twelve years, respectively, and the mean duration of the diabetes was five years.

At the beginning of the study, the mean weekly blood glucose was a high 214 mg/dl—a further indication of the overall poor control, even though urine was tested regularly. The parents and children were taught how to measure blood glucose. According to Dr. Selink, "Most children over the age of eight performed the finger pricks by themselves and found it less threatening than the administration of their insulin." The home monitoring was more difficult in the younger children, however. "The age group of three to six years has been difficult," Dr. Selink reported, "and except for especially difficult [to control] patients, we have tended to use home blood glucose monitoring only for the management of vomiting illness and other acute medical crises."

Most of the children in Dr. Selink's study were put on two insulin injections a day. "Intensive education by the medical staff, nurse educator, dietitians, and nurses was given to the patient and his or her parents. The responsibility for changing the insulin and adjusting the diet was then given to the family." (The protocols for this are given in Chapter 5.)

The patients and parents were taught to graph blood glucose levels and to keep careful records. Initially, blood glucose was measured four times a day: before breakfast, lunch, and dinner and at bedtime. The goal was to maintain blood sugar between 72 and 180 mg/dl. Once glucose was stabilized in this range, the glucose self-testing was reduced to measurements before breakfast and dinner.

"In most families," Dr. Selink reported, "the children themselves learned to adjust insulin dosage and dietary portions." Among the fifty patients, eighteen required more insulin than they had been taking before the study, thirty required less, and only two remained on the same dosage. Blood sugar control improved dramatically in all but five of the children—all teenagers who had major psychological problems. The mean blood glucose for the group dropped from 214 mg/dl to 160 mg/dl, with much fewer swings from high to low.

"As an indication of acceptance of home blood glucose monitoring, most children did not wish to go back to urine testing," Dr. Selink noted, adding, "The major benefit of home blood glucose monitoring has been the alleviation of anxiety regarding the state of diabetic control." The enhanced well-being was particularly evident among patients who had experienced frequent episodes of low blood sugar. Parents also found that home blood glucose monitoring made it easier to cope with childhood illnesses. Dr. Selink also noted that by learning to test for blood glucose, both the children and their parents gained a better grasp of the disease. Many said that for the first time, they really understood what was happening and why. As a result, they could anticipate and prevent problems; in addition, the children were less likely to rebel against their treatment.

Summing Up

Childhood diabetes is difficult for all involved. In the past, there has been a tendency to forego tight glucose control as a goal, and to concentrate instead on providing as normal a development as possible with the hope of achieving better diabetes management in adulthood. This tactic led to patterns of poor control and an increased risk of serious complications. By learning and practicing home blood glucose monitoring, a better degree of diabetes control and cooperation from both parent and child can be achieved. Studies have found that children as young as eight years of age can master the techniques involved and can also learn to adjust their own insulin and food regimens. Not only do these children achieve better glucose control, they also benefit from an enhanced sense of well-being that comes from a better understanding of the disease and a feeling of being in charge.

17

Diabetes in Adolescence

Adolescence, unquestionably one of life's most difficult periods, also raises havoc with diabetes control. The disease often first appears during or just before adolescence. The hormonal changes, growth spurt, and tremendous emotional upheavals during these crucial developmental years may be triggering factors; all make diabetes more difficult to manage. In addition, there are the very real problems caused by the teenager's normal need to declare his or her independence. A diabetic child who has coped well with the disease may suddenly rebel and go out of control in all aspects. The period can be just as trying for parents and other family members. The coping strategies adopted during these formative years will, in large measure, set the pattern for future diabetes control and adjustment. This means that a number of different needs should be recognized and met. Dr. Andrew Drexler of Rockefeller University, who specializes both in studying and in treating adolescent diabetes, summarizes the specific problems of managing the disease during these years as follows:

- The need to progress through puberty at a rate comparable with nondiabetic peers.
- The need to consume enough calories and insulin for expected growth.
- The need to resolve family conflicts involving independence.
- The need to develop normal peer-group interactions.
- The need to establish sexual identity.
- The need to make career choices.

All of these are, to varying degrees, affected by diabetes; in turn, diabetes has an effect on each.

ROLE OF HORMONAL CHANGES

Puberty is marked by hormonal changes that initiate sexual maturity and contribute to the growth spurt that is characteristic of this period of life. The sequence of events that triggers puberty is still poorly understood. It appears that, in girls at least, the percentage of body fat is a key factor. Menstruation first begins when about 17 percent of the total body weight is fat; regular ovulation starts when the portion of body fat increases to 22 percent.

Before the onset of puberty, hormonal patterns begin to change. The pituitary gland secretes small amounts of luteinizing hormone, referred to as LH, and follicle-stimulating hormone, or FSH. These are both gonadotropins, meaning they stimulate the gonads (ovaries in females and testes in males) to produce hormones and carry on their reproductive functions. Just before puberty, there are small random spikes in LH secretion; during early puberty, LH secretion, especially at night, increases. The increased production of sex hormones (testosterone and estrogen) stimulate the rapid growth characteristic of puberty as well as sexual maturity. Studies have found that these processes are delayed in diabetic children whose disease is poorly controlled. The onset of puberty is later and the children are not as likely to reach their height potential. In contrast, diabetic children who are overtreated with insulin have to compensate by eating more food to prevent hypoglycemia. As a result, they may gain too much weight and experience a premature onset of puberty. This, too, may prevent a child from reaching his or her full height potential because there is very little additional upward growth after sexual maturity.

The hormonal changes of puberty affect glucose tolerance and insulin requirements because these hormones tend to increase insulin resistance. Diabetic control also is affected by the large increase in the amount of food consumed. Anyone who has teenage children can attest to the fact that they eat huge amounts of food—the increased caloric needs are summarized in the following table. The recommended 56 calories per kilogram for a fourteen-year-old boy is more than twice the caloric requirement for a normal-weight adult. Thus, the need for additional insulin to cover the increased food consumption, coupled with the normal rise in insulin resistance resulting from hormonal changes, makes diabetes control more difficult during these years. An adolescent may need as much as 2 insulin units per kilogram during a period of rapid growth, compared with the 0.6 units per kilogram required by a healthy, normal-weight adult.

CALORIE REQUIREMENTS DURING ADOLESCENCE ACCORDING TO AVERAGE WEIGHT

Age	Males Weight (kg)	Calories (per kg)	Daily Total	Females Weight (kg)	Calories (per kg)	Daily Total
10	34	74	2,500	34	68	2,300
11	37	71	2,600	38	62	2,350
12	40	67	2,700	42	57	2,400
13	45	61	2,800	47	52	2,450
14	52	56	2,900	50	50	2,500
15	57	53	3,000	52	48	2,500
16	60	51	3,050	54	45	2,420
17	62	50	3,100	54	43	2,340
18	64	49	3,100	55	42	2,270
19	65	47	3,020	55	40	2,200

EMOTIONAL FACTORS

Of course, adolescence goes far beyond physical growth and changes; it is also marked by emotional changes and maturity. Again, diabetes can affect how well the youngster copes with the normal conflicts associated with adolescence.

Traditionally, adolescence is divided into three stages: puberty, which is marked by sexual development, growth, and more independence from parental control; middle adolescence, a period of identification characterized by development of value systems and involvement with peers; and late adolescence, a time of coping with developing personal relationships, making career choices, and finding an individual role in society.

In counseling patients and health professionals on how to help diabetic adolescents cope, Dr. Drexler stresses the special needs of each stage. For example, during early adolescence, the youngsters and parents both need reassurance that the patient is capable of assuming responsibility for managing his or her diabetes. Parents are often understandably reluctant to turn over this responsibility, especially in light of the increased difficulties in diabetes control during this period. And many adolescents harbor unspoken fears that may hinder their accepting this responsibility. For example, Dr. Drexler remarks that they are afraid the disease will in some way "interfere with their normal sexual development. These fears, which are frequently not expressed, need to be discussed and eliminated."

Many diabetic adolescents have a lowered sense of self-esteem and poor self-image, which may "interfere with the process of peer-group involvements," Dr. Drexler notes. Adolescence is a time when it is especially important to be "one of the gang" and not to appear different. Many young diabetic patients feel that their disease somehow sets them apart and keeps them from being accepted by their peers, and at this stage of life, peer approval can be perhaps more important than parental approval. Adolescent patients often react, Dr. Drexler explains, "by denying their disease or by withdrawing from situations that might reveal it. In either case, the failure to establish normal peer-group interactions may have adverse effects on the ability to develop long-term relationships later in life."

In general, four types of coping techniques or personality traits should serve as warning signs to both parents and physicians. As summarized by Dr. Drexler, these are:

1. The adolescent who is ambivalent about assuming responsibility for his or her own care. "Often this type of patient will seem a

model type of diabetic," Dr. Drexler states, "without the typical rebelliousness of adolescence." But these passive youngsters, more likely to be boys than girls, suffer a retarded ego development that is likely to persist into adulthood.

2. The openly rebellious adolescent who denies his or her illness. The major danger in this coping technique lies in a failure to follow necessary dietary and other restrictions, leading to out-of-control blood sugar. These rebellious youngsters often are rushed to the hospital in ketoacidosis, but the mistaken sense of freedom gained from defying the disease is more important than admitting he or she has a disease that is not shared by the rest of the gang.

3. The manipulative adolescent who uses diabetes to avoid normal, albeit unpleasant, situations and responsibilities. These patients also fail to assume responsibility not only for managing their diabetes, but also for school work, family obligations, and other situations common to everyone. These adolescents also may have a problem in retarded ego development.

4. The narcissistic adolescent who becomes excessively preoccupied with his or her diabetes. This youngster is likely to be very self-centered and insensitive to the feelings and needs of those around him or her.

All diabetic patients harbor some of these coping techniques, Dr. Drexler notes (as do many nondiabetics). It is when they are carried to an extreme that there is cause for worry. To counter these negative patterns, Dr. Drexler and his associates have developed a model treatment program that not only promotes better diabetes control but also fosters improved psychological growth and well-being. The program is designed to strengthen the adolescent's normal drives to acquire information and to take direct action in such a way that blood glucose control will be improved while fostering healthy emotional development. As might be expected, the program is built on the principles of self-monitoring and learning to correctly adjust insulin dosages according to blood glucose. In keeping with the peer-support concept, monthly group sessions are held with a team of health professionals, including a doctor, nurse, dietitian, and psychologist. Diabetes education is emphasized at these group sessions, but other problems also are discussed. The young people are taught to measure their own blood glucose, if they do not already do so, and how to use the information to alter insulin doses. Dr. Drexler summarizes these adjustments as follows:

1. Blood sugar is tested before and after meals and at bedtime.
2. If the glucose levels are outside the treatment goals for two consecutive days, any changes in diet or activity should be evaluated.
3. If diet and activity have been constant, insulin should be adjusted accordingly. If the problem is recurring at a specific time; for example, if the before-lunch glucose is consistently high, the insulin that is peaking at that time should be increased.
4. If overall control is poor, as indicated by high levels in all measurements, the bedtime NPH should be increased by 2 units to bring the fasting blood sugar under control. Wait another day to see if further adjustments are needed in other doses.

Program patients are asked to keep daily diet, exercise, and insulin diaries and to bring these to the group sessions. "This emphasis on self-management provides adolescents with a feeling of mastery over their disease and enhances self-esteem," Dr. Drexler says. "We emphasize slow, steady progress rather than striving for immediate control. The monthly sessions allow peers to provide suggestions for improved control." In a seventeen-month analysis of the program, Dr. Drexler and his associates found there was a steady lowering of hemoglobin A_{1C}, reflecting improved control. "Most adolescents need a period of time to adjust to their disease and its implications," Dr. Drexler cautions. This may take as long as six months, but, as Dr. Drexler notes, "Given the difficulties in dealing with diabetic adolescents, this time frame is not unreasonable."

Parental support during this period is important, but parents must be careful not to overstep certain boundaries. For example, during adolescence a patient is entitled to establish a confidential relationship with a doctor, knowing that certain information shared with a doctor or other health professional will not be reported back to parents. "This is sometimes difficult for parents to accept," Dr. Drexler says, "but the diabetic adolescent is entitled to the same confidentiality and trust as other, nondiabetic patients."

"We encourage parents to show their concern and willingness to help," Dr. Peterson explains. "At the same time, the adolescent must assume increasing responsibility for controlling the diabetes." Self-testing for blood glucose is instrumental in this process because it lets the young person see the almost immediate results of indiscretions or other activities. "Many youngsters have been told repeatedly that eating a candy bar will send blood sugar soaring, but until they actually do it and measure blood sugar before and after, it may not seem real. They can also learn to experiment with exercise and foods and then be able to anticipate certain responses and prepare for them." Self-Care physicians encourage adolescent patients to form peer groups and to exchange information.

Summing Up

Under the best of circumstances, adolescence is a difficult period for both child and parents. It can be even more difficult if the youngster has diabetes. The disease becomes harder to control because of the hormonal and physical changes of adolescence. Poorly controlled diabetes can hinder the normal developmental processes; it also can have a profound effect on emotional stability and growth. In the past, there was a tendency to downplay the need for good glucose control in the hope that the young person would eventually outgrow the rebelliousness and other negative factors. This often meant frequent hospitalizations for ketoacidosis and other complications and increased the likelihood of long-term complications. A more enlightened approach, advocated by the Diabetes Self-Care Program, involves fostering an increased sense of awareness and responsibility through self-monitoring. Aspects of life that are so important to the adolescent—increased independence and peer support and approval—are used as part of the treatment process. Studies have found that this approach not only improves blood glucose control and sets the stage for life-long management of the diabetes, but it also improves self-esteem, ego development, and emotional well-being.

18

How to Avoid Foot Problems

At one time or another, almost everyone encounters foot problems: corns, calluses, blisters, ingrown toenails, bunions, infections, or injuries from sports or other causes are but a few of the common foot afflictions. For most of us, these are relatively trivial problems that can be cured by wearing properly fitted shoes and stockings or by following common-sense hygienic practices. But to the person with diabetes, even minor foot problems can develop into serious complications, such as chronic ulcers, infection, or even gangrene, leading to amputation. Fortunately, most of these problems can be prevented, but this requires meticulous attention to preventive foot care. Patients in the Diabetes Self-Care Program are taught the principles of preventive foot care, which are summarized in this chapter; patients also are urged to see a foot specialist regularly if there are any problems, such as impaired circulation or nerve damage affecting the lower extremities.

Major Causes of Foot Problems

At least three factors make diabetic patients more vulnerable to developing foot problems:

1. The nerve damage associated with the disease reduces sensitivity, including being able to perceive discomfort and pain. Very often, a callus will form over an infected sore or ulcer—something that normally would be quite painful. But if the nerves in the feet

have been damaged by the diabetes, you may not be aware that there is a problem until it becomes an open ulcer.

2. Diabetes can cause impaired circulation, particularly to the extremities. The reduced flow of blood to the feet slows the healing process in several ways: there is an inadequate number of white blood cells to fight the infection, and the reduced supply of blood also may hinder the delivery of antibiotics to infected tissue. In addition, the poor delivery of oxygen resulting from the reduced supply of blood favors the development of microorganisms, such as anaerobic bacteria, that require oxygen-free environments. Even under the best circumstances, these anaerobic organisms are often difficult to eradicate; the problems are compounded in diabetes.

3. Poorly controlled diabetes increases susceptibility to infection, which, in turn, increases insulin resistance and makes the diabetes more difficult to control. This often results in a vicious cycle: high blood sugar increases vulnerability to infection; infection makes blood sugar even harder to control; and these further increases in blood sugar exacerbate the body's ability to fight infection. Because diabetes hinders the body's natural defenses against disease, an ordinarily trivial cut or minor injury can very quickly turn into a serious infection, including gangrene. Gangrene is more than fifty times more common in diabetic patients than in the general population.

Although infection is one of the most serious foot problems that commonly afflict diabetic patients, it is by no means the only one. People with the disease also are vulnerable to a variety of foot deformities, such as clawfoot or hammertoes. For example, damage to the motor nerves, which send messages to the muscles and thereby control movement, can lead to a weakening of the affected muscles. Muscles most commonly affected in the foot are the deep toe flexors and long extensors. In time, the muscles shrink (atrophy), causing hammertoes, an elevated arch and protrusion of the ball of the foot. These deformities increase the chance of infection and other problems because they increase the risk of calluses, the breakdown of skin, and ulcerations.

Damage to the autonomic nerves also can cause foot problems. Autonomic neuropathy may reduce the ability of glands in the skin to produce sweat. As the skin becomes overly dry, tiny cracks may develop, allowing bacteria and fungi that normally live on the skin surface to invade the underlying tissue, leading to infection.

As noted earlier, damage to the sensory nerves dulls the perception of pain; it also interferes with normal gait. Ordinarily, the contraction and relaxation of muscles in the ankle and calf help the body adjust to shifting weight while walking. Damage to the sensory nerves in the lower leg and foot hampers the body's ability to make this adjustment. As a result, a person with diabetes may develop a pounding gait, not realizing that he or she is hitting the ground too hard with each step because of the inability to feel any resulting pain. This pounding gait can eventually lead to what is known as Charcot's joints, a type of arthritic damage to the ankle and foot.

PREVENTIVE FOOT CARE

Some of the underlying causes of diabetic foot problems may be prevented by good blood sugar control. But even if the diabetes is well controlled, preventive foot care should be practiced religiously. First and foremost, this means wearing comfortable shoes that fit properly. Some people, particularly those with any kind of foot deformity or sensory problem, feel it is worth the investment to have their shoes custom-made to insure that they get a perfect fit. But there is such a wide range of sizes and styles in ready-made shoes that most people can be properly fitted. Very high heels, tight boots, and other extremes, however fashionable, are not good for anyone's feet; this is particularly true for people with diabetes. Shoes should be comfortable and made of a soft, pliable material such as leather that allows for the escape of heat and moisture. Don't wear the same pair of shoes all the time; have at least two pairs and rotate them to give each a chance to dry out between wearings. A number of foot appliances are available to accommodate bunions, hammertoes, and other deformities. However, these should be fitted by a foot specialist. Moleskin or lamb's wool may be used to prevent rubbing and to relieve pressure; but again, ask the advice of a foot specialist.

Avoid walking barefoot; going without shoes increases the risk of cuts, splinters, and other injuries. When walking on the beach or swimming in the ocean, wear protective swim sandals. But remember that sandals or open shoes do not fully protect the feet, so take extra care to avoid sharp stones or other potentially harmful objects.

Feet should be inspected carefully at least once a day, and more often if there are any problems. When breaking in a new pair of shoes, wear them for only a few hours at a time, and every now and then examine your feet for any signs of blisters, rubbing, or other irritation. If your eyesight is impaired or there are other problems that make it difficult to personally inspect your feet, ask a family member or friend to do it. Specific warning signs to look for when inspecting feet include:

- Any reddening or discoloration, blisters, corns, calluses, or other signs of foot irritation, injury, or improperly fitted shoes. Pay particular attention to the pressure points on the heel, ball of the foot, big toe, and other weight-bearing parts.
- Any blisters, cracks, signs of athlete's foot, or other infection.
- Any skin problems, such as cracking, dryness, discoloration, or other abnormal signs.
- Any abnormalities of the toenails, such as thickening, invasion into the flesh (e.g., an ingrown toenail), and discoloration.

Wash feet daily, either as a part of a daily shower or bath, or separately in a foot basin. Avoid using very hot water (test the water with an elbow or thermometer if you are unable to feel how hot it is with your feet or finger). A soft brush, foot sponge, or fine pumice stone may be used to remove dead skin tissue; however, avoid coarse pumice stones or excessive rubbing. Don't soak the feet longer than ten or twelve minutes; this may further dry out the skin. Use a mild soap, rinse thoroughly, and dry carefully, including between the toes. If the skin is dry, use a lotion containing lanolin or other lubricant. Do not use alcohol or other harsh chemicals that may damage the skin. Talcum powder may be used to prevent rubbing and to remove excess moisture from between the toes; ask a doctor before using nonprescription antifungal powders to treat athlete's foot or other fungal infection.

Corns and calluses require special attention. They are accumulations of dead skin that build up at pressure points on the foot. Most are caused by poorly fitted shoes. In diabetic patients, ulcers often develop under corns or calluses and may go unnoticed until severely infected. Any reddening or other discoloration that develops in or around a corn or callus is a warning sign to see a doctor.

Never attempt to remove a corn or callus yourself. If one is just developing, it can be softened by soaking the foot in warm (not hot) water for ten minutes and then gently scrubbing with a soft brush or foot sponge. Dry and apply a lubricating oil or lotion. The corn or callus is caused by rubbing or pressure; this should be corrected by switching shoes or using moleskin or lamb's wool to protect the affected parts of the foot. If, for example, corns are being caused by overlapping toes, lamb's wool can be used to separate them. Once the source of the pressure is removed, the corn or callus should disappear on its own. If removal of the corn or callus is advisable, it should be done by a podiatrist or other foot specialist. In any event, do not attempt to pare it yourself. Also, do not use commercial corn removers, pads, or adhesives, which contain harsh chemicals that can cause further breakdown of the skin.

Toenails are still another area of potential foot problems. Toenails are important because they offer protection to the underlying tissue. Groom them regularly, and take care to avoid damaging the surrounding tissue when trimming them. Use nail clippers or an emery board or file instead of scissors, and trim nails straight across. Cutting into the corners can cause ingrown toenails, which, in turn, can lead to infection. The cuticles should be moistened with an oil (don't use commercial cuticle removers) and then gently pushed back with an orangewood stick. In grooming toenails and feet, take special care to avoid breaking the skin. People with failing eyesight or who have coordination difficulties or other problems that make foot-grooming difficult should have someone else do it—a family member, podiatrist, or professional manicurist who is experienced in diabetic foot care.

As noted earlier, toenails should be inspected regularly along with all other parts of the foot. Any thickening of the toenail may be a sign of a fungal infection that may eventually destroy the nail. Both ingrown toenails and any thickening require a doctor's attention. Cracks in the skin surrounding the toes and any sign of inflammation or infection also should be checked by a doctor.

Although properly fitted shoes are important, pay attention also to stockings or socks. They should be absorbent and changed at least daily, or more often if needed. Don't wear stockings with holes or rough spots that may rub, and make sure that they fit properly. They should not constrict the toes, nor should they have tight elastic tops that may restrict blood flow to the feet. Also, avoid wearing garters or bands that may hinder the circulation.

Maintaining good circulation to the feet is particularly important in overall good foot care. Try to keep the feet elevated when sitting; propping them on a footstool or other low object will help prevent pooling of blood in the feet. Avoid sitting with the legs crossed at the knee and avoid sitting or standing for long periods in the same position. Exposure to temperature extremes also should be avoided.

A Word About Smoking

Smoking has a harmful effect on almost every organ system and part of the body, including the feet. A number of studies have found that cigarette smoking impairs circulation, reducing the amount of oxygen that the blood carries and also the body's ability to utilize it. Diabetic patients who smoke have an increased risk of circulatory problems, including the development of leg and foot ulcers.

Where to Go for Foot Care

Your feet should be medically inspected at least once or twice a year, and more often if there are problems. This can be done by the primary physician who oversees your entire diabetic regimen; he or she also may refer you to a podiatrist or other specialist who is experienced in diabetic foot problems. Podiatrists are medical professionals who are trained to care for feet; they handle routine grooming, corn and callus removal, and foot surgery. Extensive foot surgery, such as correction of deformities, may be referred to an orthopedic surgeon who specializes in foot problems. In any event, patients should make sure that the foot-care professional—ranging from manicurist to podiatrist or orthopedist—is experienced in dealing with the special problems posed by diabetes.

SUMMING UP

Foot problems are distressingly common among diabetic patients. However, many of these problems can be avoided by careful attention to preventive care. If infection or other problems develop, early recognition of warning signs and prompt treatment are vital since even a trivial cut or ingrown toenail can quickly develop into a life-threatening infection. You should inspect your feet daily and not hesitate to enlist the assistance of others if you are hampered by poor eyesight or other difficulties.

19

Travel and Other Potential Problems

There's no vacation from diabetes, but this does not mean that people with the disease cannot enjoy a vacation just like everyone else. Sadly, many diabetic patients are fearful of venturing far from home because they worry they will encounter an emergency situation and not be able to handle it. With proper planning, people with diabetes can safely travel to even very remote parts of the world. In fact, Dr. Jovanovic sets an example with frequent trips to parts of Eastern Europe and she offers practical advice, based on her own experiences, to Self-Care patients.

Virtually everyone crossing several time zones in a short period will experience jet lag, especially if the trip is from west to east. As we all know, it takes time for the body's internal clock to reset to local time; everything seems out of kilter for a few days. We waken in the middle of the night raring to go, and feel sleepy or hungry according to the time back home. It all has to do with circadian rhythms, the poorly understood, often overlooked internal pacemakers that control such things as the flow of hormones, fluctuations in body temperature, and even mood and ability to perform. "Circadian" means about (circa) a day—circadian systems are about twenty-four hours—and, according to a group of Harvard researchers who have studied the phenomenon, each rhythm has its own "phase relationship with respect to the environmental day–night cycle as well as with respect to each other. This internal counterpoint of rhythmic structure is remarkably stable and consistent." It is understandable, then, that suddenly traveling to a time zone several hours different from home, such as going from the United States to Europe, raises havoc with these important cycles.

People with diabetes have to be particularly attuned to circadian rhythms and adjust food and insulin intake accordingly. For example, in most people, the need for insulin is at its lowest in the early morning hours, usually between midnight and 4 A.M. But then as the flow of cortisol and "wake-up" hormones increases, the need for insulin gradually rises and is at its highest during the dawn and morning hours. Studies have found that the internal clock regulating these cycles can be reset forward or back a maximum of two hours a day, and in many people, this "range of entrainment," as the resetting process is known, is only about one hour. Still, most people on vacation want to immediately start living on the same schedule as the Romans, Londoners, Parisians, etc., and will try to ignore the fact that they are hungry, sleepy, or wide awake at the wrong times.

Some doctors advise their diabetic patients to try to maintain their at-home injection schedule, but this can create problems because it does not accommodate changes in eating and sleeping times. Also, in a week or so, the internal clock will naturally be reset to the local time. A better plan is to begin shifting the internal clock a few hours forward or backward (as the case may be) before leaving and continuing the gradual shift after arriving until the change is accomplished. Say, for example, that you are flying from California to New York, which entails a three-hour time advance. When making your reservations, ask at about what time the major meal will be served. Suppose in this case that the flight leaves at 3 P.M. and that the meal will be served about two hours later. To start making the change, you could move your normal schedule ahead one hour the day before leaving; you would take your bedtime NPH and retire earlier than usual and also get up an hour earlier the next morning. The morning insulin would be taken accordingly and breakfast and lunch would be eaten an hour ahead of your regular schedule. To make sure that the meal served on the plane fits your eating pattern, you can order from a special menu—a service provided by almost all airlines as long as they have at least twenty-four hours advance notice. Even so, Self-Care physicians urge waiting until the meal is served before taking your

Regular insulin, following the same procedure you would when eating in a restaurant.

Let's assume that you arrive at your New York destination at about 11:30 p.m. local time. Your internal clock will be an hour ahead of what it normally would be at home in California, but still two hours behind the New York time. Therefore, you should eat your bedtime snack shortly after arriving and take the bedtime NPH. By the next morning, your system should be within an hour or so of New York time. Reverse adjustments will help ease you back into your normal time when you return home. If there is going to be a seven- or eight-hour advance in time zones, for instance, you should skip an injection of NPH.

If you are traveling, say, on the evening New York-to-London flight, you would take a different approach. You would inject your before-dinner Regular insulin before eating the evening meal served on the plane. But you would skip your before-bed NPH, even though you will sleep on the plane. When you wake up, pretend you already are on London time. Before breakfast is served, take your usual NPH plus morning Regular. For the next five to seven days, you will probably need an injection of Regular insulin before lunch, since it will take a few days for your body to adjust to the time difference, and lunchtime in London will coincide with your usual early-morning rise in blood sugar.

When you return home, let's assume you will be taking a morning flight from London to New York. Take your morning NPH and Regular insulin on the plane before breakfast. Inject an appropriate amount of Regular insulin before the second airplane meal is served, and take Regular again before dinner in New York. Inject your usual before-bed NPH in New York before retiring, and you should again be on your normal schedule. But since it will take your body a few days to get used to the time difference, you should plan to monitor blood sugar carefully and adjust your insulin doses and food intake accordingly.

Self-Care physicians instruct patients to be particularly careful about self-testing their blood sugar while traveling and to make the necessary adjustments in insulin dosages and food intake to keep blood glucose normal. Patients who use an insulin pump have a special advantage when traveling because the device delivers a constant supply of basal insulin, removing the need to alter NPH injection schedules, and mealtime boluses can be handled as usual. People who rely on injections can achieve similar fine-tuning by testing blood glucose and making necessary adjustments.

OTHER TRAVEL PRECAUTIONS

When traveling, you should of course make sure that you have more than enough insulin, syringes, wipes, and other materials as well as adequate reagent strips, batteries, lancets, and other items needed for glucose monitoring. Self-Care physicians advise calculating how much you will need of each item, and then taking at least twice that. Pack these supplies in a carry-on case; not only will you have them if needed en route, you also will not risk having the insulin ruined by a temperature change in the baggage compartment or having it lost along with your bags. If you use an insulin pump, make sure that you have more than enough charged batteries. If you plan to recharge batteries while traveling, check that you have the proper current adaptor; otherwise, you will not be able to use local electrical outlets.

Of course, if the need arises, you can buy additional supplies in most countries, but they may not be sold under the same brand names or be exactly what you normally use. In any event, carry with you two or three spare prescriptions as well as a letter from your doctor stating that you have diabetes. This will help avoid problems when going through customs and other inspections for drugs. You also should wear your Medic Alert identification, which is now recognized internationally.

You can also obtain a list of doctors who specialize in treating diabetes in the city or country of destination from the American Diabetes Association, 2 Park Avenue, New York, N.Y. 10016.

In Case of Illness

Illness can strike at any time, both at home and when you are traveling; knowing what to do to control blood sugar while sick often can prevent hospitalization and speed recovery. Obviously, if you are too sick to monitor blood sugar or feel you are unable to handle the situation, you should seek prompt medical attention. If you are in a strange city and do not know a doctor there, the best course may be to go to a local emergency room.

In most illnesses, insulin needs increase. If you are vomiting and unable to eat, you may be tempted to reduce the insulin dosage. Reducing the mealtime dosage may be the proper course, but the basal dosage may have to be increased because of the increased need from the infection or stress of illness. In any event, contact a doctor. If the illness is a simple viral infection, such as a cold, you may well be able to handle it yourself. But if a bacterial infection is present, prompt treatment with an appropriate antibiotic drug is in order. Frequent self-testing of blood sugar will help guide you on dosage adjustments.

It is a good idea to have a supply of glucagon on hand for use in emergency situations. Suppose, for example, that you have taken your usual injection of before-dinner Regular insulin and then suddenly feel too ill to eat or vomit shortly after eating. An injection of glucagon will prevent an insulin reaction by providing the glucose needed to accommodate the peaking insulin.

Surgery poses special problems in diabetes management. The stress of surgery is likely to increase the need for insulin; at the same time, it is important to avoid episodes of hypoglycemia during or after an operation. Since food is withheld for a period before any scheduled operation, the usual injection schedules may have to be altered. In many instances, simply repeating the bedtime dosage of NPH in the morning before the operation will be sufficient to meet the basal needs during surgery and the immediate postoperative recovery period. Increasingly, surgeons and anesthesiologists are accepting the idea of blood sugar monitoring during the operation and postsurgery recovery period, and glucose infusions and small amounts of Regular insulin to normalize blood sugar. In emergency situations, such as an accident or emergency surgery, blood sugar monitoring and control may have to be neglected to deal with the crisis of the moment. Common sense and good judgment should prevail; diabetes control may have to be sacrificed temporarily to cope with the emergency. When this is accomplished, attention can be shifted back to normalizing blood sugar.

Patients who are unable to eat for long periods after an operation, as may be the case in gastrointestinal surgery, for example, also require special monitoring and care to maintain normal blood sugar. One solution might be to give a continuous glucose infusion along with an injection of NPH every eight to twelve hours. In many hospitals, it still takes several hours to get the results of a blood test; if the patient is well enough, he or she should be encouraged to do self-monitoring and to alert the hospital staff if the results are outside the normal range. While some doctors and hospital personnel may object to this kind of in-hospital self-care, as Dr. Jovanovic notes: "Patients have rights, even when in the hospital. Patients who have mastered self-care in an everyday setting are understandably frustrated when they realize that hospital procedures may be contrary to what they need to normalize blood sugar. Since this is such an important element in preventing or overcoming infection and in achieving a prompt recovery, patients should not hesitate to speak up if they recognize there are problems."

Undergoing dental procedures also may disrupt normal eating schedules, increase stress, and raise havoc with blood sugar control. Since diabetic patients are particularly susceptible to periodontal disease and other dental problems, both patient and dentist should know how to handle control problems that are likely to arise during dental treatment. For example, many procedures require that you not eat for varying periods of time. Suppose that gum treatments are scheduled for the morning and you are not to eat breakfast; you probably will not be able to eat lunch or a midmorning snack, either. Instead of taking your usual morning Regular insulin, you would repeat the bedtime dose of NPH and keep taking this every eight hours until you resume eating. Self-monitoring of blood sugar will indicate whether this dosage should be adjusted according to the sliding scale given in Chapter 5.

A Special Word About Medic Alert

Many diabetic patients are hesitant to tell the world about their medical problems, and in the normal course of events, there is no reason why they should. But unforeseen emergencies may arise in which you are unable to talk or communicate and yet it is vital that your diabetic condition be known. You should *always* wear prominent identification letting others know that you have diabetes and whether you are using insulin. A number of identification devices are available: the most widely used are the bracelets, necklaces, wallet cards, and other devices provided by the Medic Alert Foundation. The bracelets are particularly useful because emergency medical personnel, police officers, and others are trained to look for them. Having the traditional symbols designed into a neck pendant or other piece of jewelry may be counterproductive because it might be overlooked. New, computerized Medic Alert systems enable doctors to get your entire medical history in minutes. For more information, contact the Medic Alert Foundation International, PO Box 1009, Turlock, California 95380.

Summing Up

Many special situations may require adjustments of your normal treatment regimen to maintain good blood sugar control. Some of these are enjoyable—vacation travel to far-off places, for example— while others may involve surgery, illness, or emergencies. Being prepared in advance and knowing how to handle a variety of different situations will often minimize problems in blood sugar control. If an emergency should arise and you are unable to communicate, wearing a Medic Alert bracelet that identifies you as a diabetic patient can be life-saving.

IV

Type 2 Diabetes

20

Type 2 Diabetes

Until now, we have concentrated on type 1 diabetes, which is generally the more serious form of the disease and which also presents the greater treatment challenge. The most common form of the disease, however, is type 2 diabetes, and it would be a mistake to imply that the Diabetes Self-Care Program, or any other institution devoted to the care of diabetic patients, does not devote considerable effort to this huge segment of the diabetic population. In this chapter, we will review what is known about type 2 diabetes and also present the Self-Care Program's unique approach to self-monitoring and management of this form of diabetes.

Of the approximately ten million Americans who have been diagnosed as having diabetes, about 90 percent have type 2 diabetes; similarly, most of the estimated ten million people with undiagnosed diabetes would fall into the type 2 category. The major differences between the two types of diabetes involve the ability of the pancreas to produce insulin and the patient's tendency to develop ketoacidosis, the buildup of acidic substances in the blood as a result of the breakdown of body fat. In type 1 diabetes, the body no longer is able to manufacture its own insulin. Thus, patients with this form of diabetes must have injections of exogenous insulin. In contrast, most type 2 diabetic patients produce insulin, but the amount may be inadequate or the body may be unable to use it. Most, however, do not need to have insulin injections.

Ketoacidosis, as explained earlier, results from the body's inability to use glucose, its principal fuel, even though there may be excessive amounts of it in the blood. People with type 1 diabetes are ketosis-prone; without enough insulin, they will quickly develop ketoacidosis. In contrast, patients with type 2 diabetes have higher than normal blood glucose but do not develop ketosis, explaining why this form of the disease is referred to as ketosis-resistant diabetes.

The typical type 2 diabetic patient is middle-aged and overweight; in fact, the disease was formerly referred to as adult- or maturity-onset diabetes. Pregnancy also increases the risk of type 2 diabetes. There are exceptions, however: type 2 diabetes sometimes starts during the first three decades of life, including during childhood or adolescence, although this is somewhat unusual. It also may occur in normal-weight individuals, but again, this is not the norm.

The cause or causes of type 2 diabetes are unknown. There is often a family history of diabetes, indicating the possibility of a genetic predisposition. Sometimes the disease is triggered by a viral infection, but what role, if any, this plays in the development of the disease is unknown. Stress also can trigger type 2 diabetes; in fact, sometimes the disease occurs in people subjected to excessive stress and then disappears once the stress is resolved.

As noted, most people with type 2 diabetes produce varying amounts of insulin, which may range from higher than normal to very little. Since 80 percent or more of type 2 diabetic patients are overweight, there has been a tendency to blame obesity for development of the disease. But this appears to be an oversimplification; while excessive body fat may be the major cause in many people, it is not the only one.

Because fat tissue is somewhat insulin-resistant, people who are overweight require more insulin, meaning that the pancreas must work harder to produce it. At the same time, excessive fat tissue can increase insulin resistance, meaning the body is unable to fully use the insulin that is available. This is thought to be a factor in type 2 diabetes, but there are enough exceptions to indicate that it probably is not the only thing involved. Many recent studies have concentrated on abnormalities in the cells themselves that may prevent them from using available insulin. Insulin utilization is a complicated process that is not fully understood. Cells that require insulin have specific insulin receptors on their surface. When insulin binds to these receptors, a number of changes take place within the cell, resulting in the uptake of glucose. Studies have found that in many patients with type 2 diabetes, insulin binding is decreased, which may explain their insulin resistance. But other patients have normal insulin receptors, so it seems likely that still other factors, including pancreatic failure, may be involved. There are, for example, patients with type 2 diabetes whose pancreases produce diminishing amounts of insulin, and some may eventually develop type 1 or ketosis-prone diabetes.

DIAGNOSIS OF TYPE 2 DIABETES

Most people with type 2 diabetes have few if any warning symptoms, at least in the early stages of the disease. A suspicion of diabetes may be raised by a routine urine test showing the presence of sugar. Some patients may complain of feeling tired or thirsty. The development of secondary complications—blurred vision, lowered resistance to infections, circulatory problems, reduced kidney function, sexual impotence, or other signs of nerve damage—also may point to a possibility of diabetes.

As in type 1 diabetes, a diagnosis is confirmed by measuring blood glucose. A fasting blood glucose of 140 mg/dl or more, confirmed on two separate occasions, indicates diabetes. In borderline cases (defined as fasting blood glucose levels of 105 to 140 mg/dl), a glucose tolerance test may be ordered if there is a reasonable suspicion of diabetes; for example, a family history of the disease or any symptoms. If not, the likely course will be periodic measurement of blood glucose and steps to normalize the elevated blood sugar, such as losing excess weight and increasing exercise.

In the past, people in this borderline group were often labeled prediabetic, a classification that could be detrimental both psychologically and in terms of such things as insurance and employment. "Since a large number of people in this borderline range never go on to develop diabetes, we think it is a mistake to give them a label that indicates they will," Dr. Peterson explains. "We prefer to tell these borderline patients that they should have their blood sugar checked regularly, and that they should be aware of any changes or symptoms that may indicate development of the disease. We also outline preventive steps they can take."

TREATMENT OF TYPE 2 DIABETES

Once a diagnosis of type 2 diabetes is established, a treatment program will be designed to bring the elevated blood sugar into the normal range. Although ketoacidosis is not a danger in type 2 diabetes as it is in type 1, the basic goal of normal blood sugar applies to both types. Patients with type 2 diabetes have an increased risk of the same secondary complications that face type 1 diabetic patients. These include loss of eyesight from diabetic retinopathy, cataracts, or other disease-related causes; kidney failure; nerve damage; high blood pressure, heart attacks, strokes, and other cardiovascular disorders; impaired peripheral circulation, especially to the legs and feet; infection; and amputation. (All of these are discussed in detail in the respective chapters in Part II.) While type 2 diabetic patients may have marked hyperglycemia, most do not require insulin injections, at least in the early stages of the disease, if their pancreases are still producing adequate insulin. (An exception is the pregnant woman, whose treatment is discussed in Chapter 9.) For most of these patients, reduced food consumption and increased exercise will lower blood sugar to the normal range. If this is inadequate, drugs known as oral hypoglycemics may be prescribed.

DIETARY MANAGEMENT

Diet is a vital element in controlling both type 1 and type 2 diabetes, but most of the restrictions that people with type 1 diabetes must follow are not crucial in type 2. For example, type 2 diabetic patients do not need to worry about distributing their calories over a specific number of meals and snacks or divide them among the nutrient groups. Nor is it necessary to eat extra food to prevent an excessive lowering of blood sugar from exercise; in fact, hypoglycemia is not a problem encountered by type 2 patients unless they are taking supplemental insulin. In short, virtually all patients with type 2 diabetes can lower blood sugar, at least to some degree, by restricting food consumption. This is particularly true in overweight patients. However, as any overweight person who has repeatedly attempted to lose weight knows, cutting back on the amount of food consumed is a difficult assignment, especially when it is for life.

"The very real difficulty in sticking to a calorie-restricted diet is what makes treating type 2 diabetes so challenging," says Dr. Peterson. Scores of studies have been undertaken to devise workable dietary regimens to treat type 2 diabetes and to come up with new ways to help patients stick to them. These plans include behavior modification, hypnosis, group therapy, and peer-support groups, such as Weight Watchers. All are potentially effective, but the overall failure rate remains high. The reason is all too familiar. Dr. Jovanovic explains: "When the diabetes is first diagnosed, the patient is frightened and highly motivated. After a period of intensive dieting, sometimes in a hospital setting, the blood sugar is brought down to normal, the patient feels better, and the diabetes seems less threatening. Gradually, the person backslides, slipping back into the former eating habits. Many will starve themselves for a few days before seeing the doctor, which means that the blood sugar may be normal for the physician visit. But the diabetes certainly isn't under control."

Self-Care Program physicians have adopted a different approach. Instead of building the treatment program around a strict diet and calorie-counting, they focus on self-monitoring of blood glucose. Many doctors feel that it is not necessary for type 2 diabetic patients to do the blood tests, arguing that they do not face the same danger of ketoacidosis or hypoglycemia as type 1 patients and that they may become overly concerned and preoccupied with their diabetes. Self-Care physicians counter this by noting the high rate of failure to lower blood sugar among patients treated in the traditional manner and contrasting this with their own experience. So they teach the patients how to monitor their own blood glucose and what to do to bring it into the normal range. "This still involves eating less," Dr. Jovanovic says, "but the goals and focus are shifted from food to blood sugar." And it seems to work. Once a patient sees the effect of food on blood sugar and learns how to adjust food intake to keep blood glucose normal, compliance somehow seems easier. "We don't dwell on what a patient can or can't eat," Dr. Jovanovic says. "Our dietitians provide counseling on how to calculate calories, the basics of good nutrition, meal planning, eating habits, and other such factors. But the focus of treatment is not centered on self-denial of food; instead, it is keeping blood sugar normal. Patients who practice home blood glucose monitoring very quickly figure out how much food they can eat and not have a rise in blood sugar."

Studies have found that up to 80 percent of all type 2 diabetic patients can control their disease by diet alone, or, for sedentary people, a combination of diet and increased exercise. Exercise decreases insulin resistance, which usually is the major problem in type 2 diabetes. During exercise, the muscles burn glucose (instead of fatty acids as is the case while at rest). Regular aerobic exercise also may help lower blood cholesterol, protect against heart disease, reduce the effects of stress, and promote a sense of well-being. Thus, the exercise prescription is a very important element in the treatment program for all diabetic patients. (See Chapter 7 for a more detailed discussion.)

THE USE OF ORAL HYPOGLYCEMICS

For normal-weight people with type 2 diabetes or for those patients whose blood sugar is not adequately lowered by self-monitoring, food reduction, and exercise, oral hypoglycemic drugs may be prescribed. These drugs may be given alone or in combination with insulin. Sometimes insulin is given in the beginning to normalize blood sugar and then gradually stopped.

There are two types of oral hypoglycemics—the sulfonylureas and the biguanides. A drug called phenformin was the main biguanide used, but its sale is now banned in this country because of its potential for serious side effects, including a buildup of excessive lactic acid in the blood. The sulfonylureas, however, are widely used and are marketed under several brand names and in slightly different formulations.

The sulfonylureas were discovered during World War II by French scientists who were studying sulfa drugs. Before penicillin came into wide use, sulfa drugs (or sulfonamides) were the major antibiotics. The French researchers noted, however, that many of the mice used in their experiments were dying unexpectedly. Tests determined severe hypoglycemia as the cause of death. At the time, the more pressing need was for antibiotics to fight the infections that are so common with war injuries, so it was not until after the war that any serious attention was paid to the serendipitous discovery that sulfonamides lowered blood sugar. In the 1950s, researchers in several countries set about developing drugs from the sulfonamides that could lower blood glucose. The first such drug was introduced in Germany in 1955. It was called carbutamide and was also used briefly in this country, but was then discontinued because of its adverse side effects. In 1956, another sulfonylurea, called tolbutamide (brand name Orinase), was introduced. This was followed by chlorpropamide (Diabinese), acetohexamide (Dymelor), and tolazamide (Tolinase). Still other sulfonylureas are used in Europe and recently some of them (Glipizide and Gliburide) have become available here.

These drugs do not work in patients with type 1 diabetes, but for people whose pancreases are still producing at least some insulin, they can be effective in lowering blood glucose. It is not known exactly how the drugs work, but studies indicate that initially they stimulate the pancreas to produce more insulin. After a period of time, however, the insulin levels return to their pretreatment or even lower levels. When this occurs, the drugs' continued effectiveness in lowering blood glucose is attributed to lowered insulin resistance, resulting in a more effective use of available insulin.

The major differences among the drugs is in their duration of action. Tolbutamide is broken down in the liver and the by-products are excreted in the urine. It is a fast-acting drug with a relatively short duration of action; therefore, it should be taken two or three times a day. Acetohexamide is broken down in the liver and kidneys and also is a fast-acting drug. Its effects can be measured in one to two hours, but it has a relatively long duration of action, ranging from twelve to twenty-four hours. It is taken once or twice a day. Tolazamide is metabolized to six major compounds, three of which lower blood glucose to varying degrees. It is a relatively slow-acting drug, reaching its peak effectiveness in about seven hours, with a duration of action ranging from twelve to twenty-four hours. It also is taken once or twice a day, depending on the response in lowering blood sugar. Chlorpropamide takes the longest to act—when it is started, the effects may not be noticed for several days. It also has the longest duration of action, up to sixty hours, and it is taken once a day.

Patients on oral hypoglycemic drugs should be cautious about taking other drugs that also may lower blood sugar. For example, sulfa drugs used as antibiotics (Gantrisin, Sulfadiazine, Nefrosul, or Gantanol, among others) lower blood sugar and when taken with any of the sulfonylureas, there may be a compounded effect. Other drugs that have this effect include chloramphenicol (Chloromycetin), bishydroxycoumarin (Dicumarol), phenylbutazone (Butazolidin), oxyphenbutazone (Tandearil), and clofibrate (Atromid-S). To avoid possible drug interactions, always let your doctor know about any medications, including over-the-counter or nonprescription drugs, that you are taking before starting any new drug.

Since 1969, there has been a continuing medical and scientific controversy over the use of oral hypoglycemic drugs, based on results of the University Group Diabetes Program (UGDP) study. This study, started in 1961, was intended to assess the effectiveness of the oral hypoglycemic drugs and to learn more about the natural course of type 2 diabetes. Study volunteers, all of whom had been diagnosed as having type 2 diabetes for at least one year, were followed for five years. The patients were recruited from twelve university-affiliated clinics. They were divided into four groups: one group took tolbutamide twice a day, one a placebo, and the other two groups were treated with insulin: one a standard dosage and the other a minimal dose of 10 to 16 units of an intermediate insulin. The controversy arose when tolbutamide was abruptly discontinued because it appeared to increase the risk of heart attacks.

Ever since, researchers have argued that the results of the UGDP were invalid because of flaws in the original study design. Some of the patients had been recruited from cardiology clinics, and may have had serious heart disease when they entered the study. At the time, there was no effective way to measure long-term blood glucose control, so it was not known whether this was a factor. Also, the overall mortality figures between the placebo- and tolbutamide-treated groups did not differ. Later studies have not found an increase in heart attacks among patients taking tolbutamide.

Today, most experts, including Self-Care Program physicians, agree that high blood sugar probably poses a greater long-term risk than the use of oral hypoglycemic drugs. If, after a few months of diet and exercise therapy, blood glucose remains over 200 mg/dl, most doctors now agree that a sulfonylurea should be prescribed. The drug may be discontinued if the patient loses enough weight and increases exercise enough to normalize blood glucose.

USE OF INSULIN IN TYPE 2 DIABETES

In some patients, particularly those who are extremely obese, sulfonylureas may not be enough to normalize blood sugar. For these patients, the regimen may be supplemented by insulin injections. Some type 2 patients are initially given insulin to lower blood glucose and are then weaned to a sulfonylurea. Patients using insulin alone or a combination of insulin and oral drugs must learn to self-test for blood sugar.

Many type 2 patients never need insulin; some, however, experience increasing pancreatic failure and eventually require an insulin therapy regimen similar to that of type 1 patients. Again, self-monitoring of blood sugar is an important tool in determining whether such treatment is needed.

Summing Up

Type 2 diabetes, the most common form of the disease, differs from type 1 in several important respects, especially in the area of insulin production and use and the tendency to develop ketoacidosis. The majority of type 2 patients are overweight, and their diabetes can be treated by reducing food intake and increasing exercise. This has proved very difficult for large numbers of patients, especially those who find it hard to stick to a diet. Self-Care Program physicians have found that self-monitoring of blood sugar is an important incentive to these patients because it shifts the emphasis from food to normalizing blood sugar.

If blood sugar cannot be sufficiently lowered by diet and exercise, oral hypoglycemic drugs may be prescribed. And for some patients, insulin also may be needed.

Afterword

The concepts in this book represent an important beginning. New goals have been defined in terms of blood glucose levels for persons with diabetes and tools and skills have become available to achieve these goals.

Yet normal blood glucose is not achieved 100 percent of the time by all patients with diabetes. The concepts in this book will help to maintain optimum health until even better tools come along. And what does the future hold?

It is now possible to manipulate the immune system so that people who are in the early stage of type 1 diabetes may not end up losing all of their insulin-producing cells. Furthermore, certain viruses that cause diabetes are being characterized with the hope of creating a vaccine to prevent some forms of the disease.

Insulin delivery will become easier. Pumps are becoming smaller, safer, and easier to handle. Computers will soon be available to help with insulin dosage decision-making. Linking the computers with the pump and a glucose sensor will allow the whole system to be implanted some day.

It is also now possible to culture the beta cells that make insulin and get them to respond appropriately in the test tube. Problems of injection of transplanted islets are being overcome and therefore transplanting islet tissue will soon be possible as treatment for diabetes.

These are times of tremendous hope for people with diabetes. Yet the best hope remains to maintain blood glucose levels as close to normal as possible and stay as healthy as possible in order to most benefit from the coming developments.

Lois Jovanovic, M.D.
Charles M. Peterson, M.D.

Glossary

ACIDOSIS: An increase in the acid content of the blood. In diabetes, ketoacidosis occurs when the body cannot use glucose and starts breaking down fat, producing the acidic buildup that increases the ketone bodies in the blood and urine.

ADRENALINE (ALSO CALLED EPINEPHRINE): A hormone secreted by the adrenal glands, which are situated above the kidneys. Adrenaline is released when the body perceives danger, triggering the fight or flight response. Among other things, adrenaline raises blood glucose levels and therefore increases resistance to insulin.

ALPHA CELLS: Cells in the pancreas that produce glucagon, the hormone that stimulates the production of glucose.

AUTOIMMUNE RESPONSE: A disorder in which the immune system produces antibodies against the body's own tissues. Some researchers think that the destruction of the pancreatic beta cells that occurs in type 1 diabetes may be caused by an autoimmune response.

BASAL INSULIN: Constant amount of insulin required for basal metabolism, or to provide energy needed for basic body processes and functions.

BETA CELLS: Insulin-producing cells located in the islets of Langerhans in the pancreas.

CARBOHYDRATES: Dietary starches and sugars, which are the body's major source of energy. Diabetes is characterized by an inability to properly metabolize carbohydrates.

CATARACT: An abnormal clouding or opacity of the eye's lens.

CHARCOT'S JOINTS: Arthritic damage to ankle and foot joints caused by diabetic damage to the nerves, leading to a heavy step or pounding gait. Named for the French physician who first described the phenomenon.

CHOLESTEROL: A fatty substance found in the brain, nerves, liver, blood, and bile. Cholesterol is not easily broken down, and an overabundance may lead to atherosclerosis, a buildup of fatty deposits in the artery walls.

CORNEA: The transparent membrane that protects the outer surface of the eye.

CREATININE: The waste product of protein breakdown that is found in normal urine. Excessive breakdown of the body's muscle tissue, such as that which occurs during starvation or uncontrolled diabetes, leads to elevated creatinine in the urine.

DIURETIC: A drug or agent that reduces the accumulation of body fluid, which in turn increases the volume of urination.

FASTING BLOOD GLUCOSE: Level of blood sugar as measured after a period of fasting, such as before eating in the morning.

FIBER: The indigestible plant material also known as roughage.

GESTATIONAL DIABETES: Diabetes that starts during pregnancy and disappears after delivery.

GLOMERULUS: The kidney part that filters from the blood the liquid containing waste material and nutrients.

GLUCAGON: The hormone produced and secreted by the alpha cells of the pancreas gland. It raises the level of blood sugar. In diabetic patients, glucagon counteracts hypoglycemic reactions by mobilizing glycogen, or stored sugar.

GLUCOSE (DEXTROSE OR BLOOD SUGAR): The most common monosaccharide (simple sugar) and the main source of energy for humans.

GLUCOSE METER: Device used to calculate level of blood glucose using chemical reagent strips; an important tool in home blood glucose monitoring.

GLYCOGEN: The form in which glucose is stored in the liver. Glycogen is easily converted into glucose.

GLYCOSURIA: Presence of sugar in the urine and a frequent sign of diabetes.

GLYCOSYLATION: The process that links glucose with another substance, such as hemoglobin.

HAMMERTOES: Foot deformity in which the toe is permanently foreshortened and cannot be straightened. May be caused by a shortening of the muscle, improperly fitted shoes, or congenital defect. Hammertoes are common in diabetic patients who have impaired circulation and nerve function in the feet, leading to muscle atrophy.

HEMOGLOBIN: The oxygen-carrying component of red blood cells.

HEMOGLOBIN A_{1C}: Hemoglobin in which a glucose molecule is permanently attached to the two beta chains found in normal hemoglobin. The amount of hemoglobin A_{1C} reflects the average blood sugar over a six- to eight-week period.

HYPERGLYCEMIA: An excessive level of blood sugar.

HYPERTENSION: Higher than normal blood pressure. Hypertension is a major risk factor for heart attacks and kidney failure; it is also the leading cause of strokes.

HYPOGLYCEMIA: A deficient level of blood sugar.

INSULIN: The hormone produced and secreted by the beta cells of the pancreas gland that is essential to metabolism, particularly of carbohydrates, but also of protein and fat. A failure to produce or inability to use insulin results in diabetes.

INSULIN PUMP: Portable device consisting of an insulin reservoir, power source, computer, tubing, and needle to provide a continuous infusion of insulin. The pump also can be programmed to deliver larger amounts of insulin as needed to cover food or counter hyperglycemia.

INSULIN RESISTANCE: Failure of the body to effectively use available insulin. Infection, stress, pregnancy, and obesity are among the factors that increase insulin resistance.

ISLETS OF LANGERHANS: The groups of alpha and beta cells in the pancreas.

KETOACIDOSIS: The buildup of ketone bodies in the blood and urine. (Also see Acidosis.)

KETONE BODIES: Chemical compounds formed during fat metabolism. Components are highly acidic and include acetone, acetoacetic acid, and beta-hydroxybutyric acid.

KETONURIA: Presence of ketones in the urine, a sign of ketoacidosis. Can be measured with reagent strips or tablets.

LASER BEAM: A beam of concentrated light that can be controlled to sever, eliminate, or fuse body tissue. Laser beam surgery is used to treat eye disorders, such as diabetic retinopathy.

LENS: The transparent tissue of the eye that focuses rays of light to form an image on the retina.

LEUKOCYTES: The white blood cells, which are instrumental in fighting infection. Patients with poorly controlled diabetes have abnormally functioning white blood cells, making them more susceptible to infection.

LIPID: A fatty substance, such as cholesterol or triglycerides.

LIPODYSTROPHY (ALSO LIPOATROPHY): The scientific term for atrophy, or shrinking, of fat tissue. An example is the hollow places that sometimes form where insulin has been injected into the fatty tissue underlying the skin.

LIPOHYPERTROPHY: Buildup of fatty tissue that causes the bulges that sometimes form at insulin injection sites.

LIPOPROTEINS: The compounds of lipids and proteins that carry cholesterol in the blood. Three types of lipoproteins are very low-density lipoproteins (VLDL), which carry mostly triglycerides, and low-density lipoproteins (LDL) and high-density lipoproteins (HDL), which carry cholesterol. A high level of LDL cholesterol is associated with an increased risk of atherosclerosis and cardiovascular disease, while a high level of HDL cholesterol is believed to protect against heart disease.

MYOPATHY: A disease affecting the muscles.

NEPHRONS: The filtering units of the kidney. Each nephron contains a glomerulus and tubules.

NEPHROPATHY: Disease affecting the nephrons.

NEUROPATHY: A disease affecting the nervous system.

OPPORTUNISTIC INFECTION: Disease caused by a microorganism that is normally harmless, but which can cause a serious infection in patients whose defenses are weakened by other diseases, such as diabetes or immune-system deficiencies.

OPTIC NERVE: The fiber that transmits optic impulses from the retina to the brain.

ORAL HYPOGLYCEMIC AGENT: A substance taken by mouth to lower blood glucose levels by stimulating either increased production or utilization of insulin.

PANCREAS: The gland located in back of the upper midabdomen, in which insulin, glucagon, and digestive enzymes are produced. A failure of the pancreas to produce adequate insulin for carbohydrate metabolism leads to elevated blood glucose and diabetes.

PHOTOCOAGULATION: The type of laser surgery that destroys some of the tiny aneurysm or excessive capillaries that are characteristic of diabetic retinopathy.

PITUITARY GLAND: The master gland located at the base of the skull. It controls many of the other glands in the body by producing and secreting hormones.

PLACENTA: The circular fleshlike tissue through which substances are exchanged between mother and fetus.

PLATELETS: The components of blood that form clots to stop bleeding. People with diabetes often have more active platelets and therefore form blood clots more easily.

PROLIFERATIVE RETINOPATHY: Overgrowth of fragile new blood vessels on the retina that may leak blood into the eyeball.

PROTEINS: Organic compounds made up of particles called amino acids. Proteins are essential to maintaining and building body tissue; they also may be converted to glucose to provide energy, but more slowly than carbohydrates.

PROTEINURIA (ALSO ALBUMINURIA): Protein in the urine, a common sign of kidney disease.

REAGENT STRIPS: Chemically treated strips that are used in measuring blood glucose. A drop of blood is placed on the strip, which then is interpreted either visually by noting color change or in a glucose meter.

RETINA: The layered lining of the eye that contains light-sensitive receptors (the rods and cones) and conveys images to the brain.

RETINOPATHY: An injury or disease of the retina.

TUBULE: The kidney part that removes the waste products from the liquid separated from the blood by the glomerulus for excretion as urine and returns the nutrients and other useful products to the circulation.

TYPE 1 DIABETES (ALSO CALLED INSULIN-DEPENDENT, KETOSIS-PRONE, OR JUVENILE-ONSET DIABETES): The diabetes type that is generally (but not always) acquired in the first three decades of life and that is characterized by failure of the pancreas to produce insulin.

TYPE 2 DIABETES (ALSO CALLED NONINSULIN-DEPENDENT, KETOSIS-RESISTANT, OR MATURITY-ONSET DIABETES): The diabetes type that usually (but not always) occurs in adulthood, generally after the age of forty. The pancreas still produces insulin, although the amount may be insufficient to meet the body's needs, or the body may be resistant to the insulin, which may be present in even higher than usual amounts. Type 2 diabetes is often treatable by reduced intake of food, especially in obese patients, and exercise. Sometimes oral hypoglycemic agents or insulin also are required.

VITREOUS HUMOR: The jellylike substance that is found between the lens and the retina and that supports the interior parts of the eye.

Appendix

FOR ADDITIONAL INFORMATION

A number of organizations and educational programs devoted to helping people with diabetes are located throughout the United States. More information about these programs may be obtained by contacting the following:

American Diabetes Association, Inc.
2 Park Avenue
New York, N.Y. 10016
Phone: (212) 683-7444

The Juvenile Diabetes Foundation
23 East 26th Street
New York, N.Y. 10010
Phone: (212) 889-7575

National Diabetes Information Clearinghouse
Box NDIC
Bethesda, Md. 20205
Phone: (301) 468-2162

Diabetes Education Foundation
215 Sandringham Road
Rochester, N.Y. 14610
Phone: (716) 385-3601

Joslin Diabetes Center
One Joslin Place
Boston, Mass. 02215
Phone: (617) 732-2400

Sansum Medical Research Foundation
2219 Bath Street
Santa Barbara, Calif. 93105
Phone: (805) 682-7638

Selected Bibliography

Brown, Mark J., and Arthur K. Asbury. "Diabetic Neuropathy," *Annals of Neurology*, Vol. 15, No. 1, pp. 2–12, January 1984.

Burrow, Gerard N., et al. "A Case of Diabetes Mellitus," *New England Journal of Medicine*, Vol. 306, No. 6, pp. 340–41, February 11, 1982.

Davidson, Mayer. *Diabetes Mellitus: Diagnosis and Treatment.* New York: Wiley Medical, 1981.

Fredholm, Nancy Zilinsky. "The Insulin Pump: New Method of Insulin Delivery," *American Journal of Nursing*, Vol. 81, No. 11, pp. 2024–34, November 1981.

International Workshop on Insulin (proceedings of), sponsored by Juvenile Diabetes Foundation, May 4–6, 1978, New York City.

Jovanovic, Lois. *Your Guide to a Healthy, Happy Pregnancy.* Indianapolis: Bio-Dynamics, 1981.

Jovanovic, Lois, Maurice Druzin, and Charles M. Peterson. "Effect of Euglycemia on the Outcome of Pregnancy in Insulin-Dependent Diabetic Women as Compared with Normal Control Subjects," *The American Journal of Medicine*, Vol. 71, No. 12, pp. 921–27, December 1981.

Jovanovic, Lois, and Charles M. Peterson. "Home Blood Glucose Monitoring," *Comprehensive Therapy*, Vol. 8, No. 1, pp. 10–20, January 1982.

————. "Management of the Pregnant, Insulin-Dependent Diabetic Woman," *Diabetes Care*, Vol. 3, No. 1, pp. 63–68, January–February 1980.

————. "Modern Monitoring and Management of the Diabetic Pregnant Patient," in *Modern Management of High-Risk Pregnancy*, Niels H. Lauersen, editor. New York: Plenum, 1983.

————. "Optimal Insulin Delivery for the Pregnant Diabetic Patient." *Diabetes Care*, Vol. 5, No. 3, Part 2, pp. 24–37, May–June 1982.

Linn, Lawrence S., and Charles E. Lewis. "Attitudes Toward Self-Care Among Practicing Physicians," *Medical Care*, Vol. 17, No. 2, pp. 183–90, February 1979.

Moore-Ede, Martin C., et al. "Circadian Timekeeping in Health and Disease, Part 1," *New England Journal of Medicine*, Vol. 369, No. 8, pp. 469–76, August 20, 1983.

Overweight and Diabetic. New York: CME Communications Inc., 1979.

Plamberg, Paul, et al. "The Natural History of Retinopathy in Insulin-Dependent Juvenile-Onset Diabetes," *Ophthalmology*, Vol. 88, No. 7, pp. 613–18, July 1981.

Peterson, Charles M. *Take Charge of Your Diabetes: A New Approach to Self-Management.* South Bend, Ind.: Just Mailings, 1982.

————, ed. *Diabetes Management in the '80s.* New York: Praeger, 1982.

Schade, David S., and R. Philip Eaton. "Insulin Delivery—Today's Systems, Tomorrow's Prospects," *Drug Therapy*, Vol. 9, No. 5, pp. 47–55, May 1981.

Tamborlane, William, et al. "Outpatient Treatment of Juvenile-Onset Diabetes with a Preprogrammed Portable Subcutaneous Insulin Infusion System," *The American Journal of Medicine*, Vol. 68, No. 2, pp. 190–96, February 1980.

Index

Atheromas, 194, 197
Atherosclerosis
and blood clots, 123, 125
and cholesterol buildup, 75, 123
and insulin, 198
and platelet abnormalities, 197
Athletes, and insulin needs, 51, 52
Atrophy, 232
Autoimmune disorders, and
diabetes, 6
Autonomic nervous system, and
diabetes, 202
Autonomic neuropathy
cardiac arrest from, 203
effects of, 202, 232–33
and foot problems, 232–33
Axons, 203

Banting, Dr. Frederick G., 4, 46–
47, 48
Barron, Dr. Moses, 46
Basal insulin
calculating for insulin pump, 139,
143
and exercise, 143
function of, 138
needs in the morning, 140–41
Best, Dr. Charles H., 4, 46, 47, 48
Biguanide drugs, 252–53
Blindness, and diabetes, xiii
causes of, 187, 190
from proliferative retinopathy,
190
Blisters, 231
Blood cholesterol, 75, 76
See also Cholesterol
Blood clots
and atherosclerosis, 123, 125

causes of, 197
reducing risk of, with exercise,
125
Blood glucose, 4
carbohydrate conversion to, 4,
54, 75, 83
conversion of nutrients to, 83
fat conversion to, 83
high. *See* Hyperglycemia
and insulin, 4
low. *See* Hypoglycemia
protein conversion to, 4, 54, 76,
83
Blood glucose levels
and breakfast, 85–86
charting own, 35–39
example of patient charting, 39–
44
and exercise, 126, 131–33
measuring own, 31, 32–34
and red blood cells, 32
rise of, and infection, 211–12
and stress, 183, 184
Blood lipids. *See* Lipids
Blood sugar levels. *See* Blood
glucose levels
Bolus doses of insulin
function of, 138
for insulin pump, 139–40, 145–
46
Brain, and glucose, 4
Breakfast, 84–86
and blood glucose levels, 85–86
high-protein, 85
and insulin adjustment, 85–86
low-carbohydrate, 85
Brown, Dr. M. J., 206
Brown, Dr. W. Virgil, 194, 195